INDEX

copyright © peter sotos 1998

ONE

"Sometimes, I try to think about what is going to happen to me. Not when I'm dead, but when I'm dying. I'm scared. I get lonely at night. I want my mother to be here with me because I feel so vulnerable. I get panicky when I stop breathing. It's so claustrophobic, if you stop breathing. There's no treatment for me. If I walk in with pneumonia, they're not going to treat it. When I die, I'll die within a week. At this point, I'm so far along that I might wake up some morning with only two more days to live. I do want to be made comfortable. I want as much medicine as I need, to keep the pain away."
(PEOPLE WITH AIDS, Nicholas & Bebe Nixon, Godine, 1991)

"I'm finding that AIDS seems to have taken some of the fun out of washroom sex. People just don't ....the washrooms don't seem to be as crowded as they used to be and not as much activity is going on and they don't seem to be as fun now. There's a lot less sucking going on ....it's mostly, I think, mutual masturbation."
(URINAL, John Greyson, Art Metropole, 1993)

"Imagine the difference in gay men's lives if

we knew beyond any reasonable doubt that oral sex was as safe as plugging in a toaster. Talk about news you can use! Then again, imagine the potential number of lives saved if we learned otherwise but in the process discovered factors that can minimize the risk. The problem is that nobody anywhere is working on the question."
("Oral Arguments", Gabriel Rotello, ADVOCATE, Oct. 17, 1995)

"Call me wigger, call me a race-traitor, call me a self-loathing homosexual: I'll just tell you that you are jealous. I'm just starting to explore the ways in which one can be white and not-quite white, gay and not quite-gay, but the only thing I've learned for sure is that people don't seem to understand. But damn. You should see my trade.
     For whatever reason, I am slipping farther and farther into banjee, and it is perhaps fitting to write in the first anniversary issue of DIRTY that I have moved from one of those passable guys who gets to suck the dicks of cute boys getting off the subway at Delancy Street into one of the boys who gets his dick sucked."
(DIRTY, Chris Leslie ed., Volume 2, issue 1)

"I have developed a detailed three page questionnaire which delves into the intimate experiences of exceptionally well-endowed men. I want to find out what sort of locker comments they have encountered, how their partners react when they first see their size, and how they have coped with ill-fitting

condoms, briefs, athletic supporters, and trousers. The men who qualify for this study must measure at least 9" from the top when erect (which means that less than 1 in 100 men will be able to participate). For that reason, I need your help. If you know of any man – straight, gay, black, white, young, old – who qualifies, please let me know."
(THE HORSEMEN'S CLUB, Gary M. Griffin, Added Dimensions, 1992)

"I have had a very satisfying life and can fondly recall many of the special outstanding cocks I've sucked over the years, like the one that shot the biggest load, the butch I thought was 'straight' but wanted to be finger-fucked while getting blown, the rough trade type that insisted on calling my mouth his favorite 'pussy', the one that wanted me to hold still while he 'fucked' my mouth, and the fattest one I ever sucked (I'm not a size freak but this one was so fat with such an unbelievably large head that I can never forget it)."
(SKIN, Boyd McDonald ed., Bright Tyger, 1988)

"The essence of fucking, to me, is not penetration per se, but trust: I trust you to be gentle (or rough, or whatever), I trust you to make me feel good, I trust you enough to want your cum up my ass. Wearing a condom negates those feelings, for me, and leaves the act as a simple in-and-out act of penetration. If that's all I want, I can use a dildo. No, I want a man – but not a Negative any longer, not a man who's scared of the juices of my body. The Negative world is defined by fear, ours by

pleasure – and it takes another Positive to treat me with the abandon for which sex was invented."
("Exit The Rubberman", Scott O'Hara, STEAM, volume 3, issue 3)

If I crouch down – down to that low level – I can hear – I can fucking feel – the drop inside your skull. I can see and touch and cum all over your masturbating little fingers, your self hatred and ripped apart mouth hole.

That open mouth and pushed flat tongue, those wide open eyes and burning blush are hardly temporary faggot. This is what you smell like. This is what you've become, what you've grown up into.

Back to your hole.

Do you like the cock you get?

With your face stinking like everyone and your wetness and drool, the inside of your head repeating details of hollow mouth, frenetic violent rut, swallow and suck and throat. Pushed up against a hole cut in a cheap wall, in a bathroom or a peepshow or a faggot ghetto club designed exclusively for exactly this, any sliding fat hard cock in your face for – what – a couple minutes will not only do but be perfect. A perfect fit.

Make him cum.

Take him all the way.

All the way in.

Make him cum into you. Onto you. By your best sex giving, sex sucking, sex being efforts.

It was a very thick around cock, and long. Hung down weight. Pointed, wrinkled, dead pink and tired. Naturally, it belonged to a thin boy of about, say, twenty-two or so. He wore white boxer shorts just barely shoved down around his thighs with his meaty balls flopped heavily above the elastic waist band. His hand, at first, hid the head of his cock as he stroked his meat using that rough sort of tease and squeeze technique common to men of that size. Cupped the head and pushed and pulled by squashing his fist around and back and out and in. Through the hole in the wall you spied his darkened ruddish face, glasses and sex stupid stare. Slightly drawn, rough skin, messy hair; a little too thin for Chicago.

He reached over and tapped first.

Not hard yet, you simply brushed your hand across your crotch to show bulge and interest. Tap back.

He pulled his face away and backed up to show you the half hard-on unencumbered by fist. Wobbly and long and grey with a tight smooth well defined head. He pushed it through.

Your fingers felt its weight from underneath its languid heft. Pulled it. Wrapped a fist around it and tugged. He responded by pushing up closer to the wall and sticking his cock right up to the stem, flattening his balls and pubics up against his side of the wall.

Very thick. Very long. Getting harder.

His meat was sticky. Tacky. He had been in the booth already when you entered yours. Spit had dried on his cock so your hand, your fingers, your palm, felt its flesh snap and mat as you measured, lifted and squeezed. It would smell like someone else's mouth. It would taste like someone else's mouth – their hot tongue, their dry spittoon gums and throat, the red space open inside their head while they try to keep from biting and swallowing and drooling. His cock wanted another face. He pushed harder towards the wall. He wanted another head to fuck. A motion in his ass, a pull in his balls, a rubbing and brushing and washing blank around his cock flesh as he stared at a wooden partition trying to guess what that last stroke was: your fist, your mouth, your wet sliding tongue, you could bend over and wrap your asshole around that hard-on now and let him drive long into your body, into your gut, up inside your shitting sucking works.

    How many before you. How long would it take him to get that meat at full pointed quaking attention. Full up animal. How long would you have to work at it, love it, how long did you want to spend. Tasting his flesh, like warm skin, like a scab or a booger when you're just a child, and spongy head and pumping cells that stopped sliding and bending while you pinned your whole fucking existence on that fat fucking hard-on. Spitting and wetting it down and stroking it up and staring at it, at your work, at what you want. Hard and blood rushed and slimy and ready to cum so you poke your pointing tongue into that hole on the end of that stretched pink smooth helmet to taste and search for the body inside of that beast. Lap tickle eat those hairy heavy balls. His curly black hair patch all wirey and coarse and matted, his vein and bumps and tightness, his motion, his responses, his cum inside someone else's mouth, asshole, cock, AIDS.

    You suck it. You bend over and suck it. Swallow and deep throat it. Tongue the bottom of it and eat his meat inside your crowded panting head. Swallow someone else's gut. Some other slave dirty fuck's filthy rubber on someone else's filthy pissing dick.

Pre-cum. Inside that hole, down his thick long stem into his balls around his nerves, his stomach, intestines, out down his prostate and flexed into his skinny little pinched dirty prune shitted asshole.

Turn around. I want to suck your ass.

That dried spit taste is yours now. All you have now is burning you; hot and wet and transformed like a fat ugly dog lapping and eating someone else's greasy waste, anyone's hole. Sniffing up a stranger.

Do you think you can cum again?

As you settle into animal rhythm.

I'll know when you're ready.

Do you want to suck that up too?

Dogs don't know better. Dogs don't know anything. Dogs are made for this.

Bugs.

Lice. Can crabs scurry up a dick into a hot mouth, does your spit, your fat lips slick them out of that black pubic nest and do you eat them along with the yeast and stink and flesh and spit and stick.

What comes first: the loser or the loss?

You have to be this way, don't you?

Who fucked you up like this?

There's a certain strain of glory hole slob that likes to show off its prowess. You feel this sort of primped hog on the end of your pisshole and it's bad enough. To watch him work on someone else is worse. PR terms like homophobia and intolerance mean nothing next to the, very sexual if you like, urge to see the cocksucker hurt, bleeding and crying. There is a sense of craft that reads mindless and weak and, in its self-importance and singularity, comes across as confrontational. Designed, as it is here, to entice. Men look hideous in this position. As do women. But if a vagina provokes an urge to mutilate like a stomach worm provokes an urge to vomit, then a cocksucker – his head cracked open like the best cunt he never had – deserves to know exactly what it is he's playing at. Which only you can explain.

    Came in here looking for a pig.

    Came in here to celebrate all that is unfair. All the little rats that can't keep their jaws above the rushing sewer black water. The rats that drilled their ways out of their little concrete holes – coming out, declaring themselves in bright white chiffon lights and back pats, hugs and angry parental cartoons – and up into the bottom of the world. Sweaty short matted dysgenic rodent coats scraped and bloodied and patched, pointy evil little stubby teeth chipping and digging and ragging on the fat bloated worn brethren in front of them: blocking their way, their turn at the hole; at the drop feeder. The grosser ones who don't know their sickness. The ones who clean up, pay and lie. Mice, just as dirty and infected and rotting, being chewed slower and even more painfully by the cramped cages it keeps dropping itself into.

    Came in here to look down. To lift up my shoe and see the cum on the floor turn to a small stain. Saw the kleenex and rubbers and thick wet puddles of dead waste – piss, cum with parasites, infectors and drugs. The chlorine stink that bites less and less from the nigger's $5.00 an hour mop and more and more from the spent cocks of cock hungry mama's boys.

    Do you work here, or just hanging around?
    I help out.

He's got two very clear sores – like little warts, one right on top of each other, or rather, right next to each other like a deep inverted staple gun scar – on the top of his long cock.

Suck it.

He's already hard. And standing straight up in the air like some showered teenager who can't wait for a kiss or a piss or a pat. And doesn't really know the difference.

His speech has that irritating, slightly southern lisp. That affected fag or traditional white trash slide.

He stuck his finger through next.

He licked the head of my dick in even concentric circles and beat the shaft so quickly and so steadily that cumming was strictly relief. Which is all it ever is, probably.

I can tell when I cum into someone's mouth, when all I can see is the wood in front of me. My cock twitches and expels and the mouth clamps tighter. In the best cases. I can feel the back of its throat, a bit busy because of the orgasm, but this wet warm roughness is there. And you draw back clean. He wasn't going to lick the cum off the end, just swallow it straight down.

I could give it AIDS if, I hear, his gums are bleeding or he has herpes or a cold sore inside that head cunt.

He's still beating off. Still working it. Usually they cum at the same time, or before, I think.

"You belong to me now," he says as I button up and turn to walk out.

What does this waste do? What goes on in that house at night; let alone in his brain. In his dingy little apartment. His sick little life, his lonely faggy words.

      I see him sitting in a chair – that his mother bought him a long time ago – just staring off into space. His right leg has gone from twitching to pounding. Uneven nerves constantly shaking and tapping as he just forgets himself if he can. Nervous about what's happening, what's not happening and what, exactly, he's not doing right now.

      TV is boring. Cable is paid for and wasted. He searches the channels for sex scenes. Insulting stupid plots only designed to show fake tits once in awhile. The news reports have all been used up between 4:00 and 7:00 and he just can't fucking sit through the same fucking things again. His CDs are all the same. The food is all the same.

      He's just watching, thinking, imagining what his bed would feel like if he could sleep. If he felt like sleeping rather than just having a decision made for him. His leg shaking all the way through his hips into his stomach.

      It's not me that's wrong.

      All cocks are the same. Size queens try so hard to put personality where it doesn't belong. Everyone is flat as soon as they walk, cock first, through the door.

      After all these years trolling around for mouths to fuck and cocks to suck, the part of the act he hates the most is seeing what pig comes attached to the meat.

      At the holes – better than the fake baths that barely exist or the tea room pop-ups or faggot bars; he never goes home with anyone anymore – he's grown disgusted with those games. He doesn't even worry about cops anymore. If he's looking to feed, he just stuffs his wobbly soft cock through and waits to be serviced. He's yet to be arrested or turned down outright. No matter how limp or unwashed for how long or scabby he is. Most of the time the lunching breaks down before a full hard-on is reached. And if he's looking for meat, he refuses to bend and peer. He just juts his finger through the dark hole and drops and licks and sucks hard when served. Like a zoo. Size is for the queens and dykes. For the new boys and the lost. All the same thing.

He doesn't want to know what he got: just some penis. Some part of a man who means less than shit. Some sex act. Some sex. Some internal confusion. A fat long thick one that tastes like some greaseball's fist or a short stub, uncircumcised, that sucks hard too quick and cums too politely. Tall and thin, and slow to get hard should read HIV positive, because of its popularity. Fat ones mean laborers. Beer guts and cake guts and shy locker room wife problems. Too many tasted like someone else's dirty breath. And bad manners.

T-shirts he'd see. Bad jackets. Suits. Stained and shit lumped underwear. Some rude motherfuckers who'd put condoms on before slipping it through. Ask, cunt. Let me see you unwrap the thing before I tap you back. Push you back into your – suburban – hole.

Size is nothing now. Taste and smell are irritants. The place he goes to the most reeks worse than any nigger plug package anyway: the fat fuck who runs the joint weighs some four hundred pounds and can barely be moved to give change for the slots these days. His huge black nigger dollop neck is strangled with tumours. If not thick black keloid knife scars.

Any cock comes through, he sucks. Any

mouth that shoves itself into the wall, first, he fucks.

That belly motherfucker needs an iron lung. His wheezes and farts and sloth are what's really at root here. And his disdain or indifference or capitalism, nigger-style, just rots everything in slow time. It's his stink that covers everything.

Stick your balls through.

Nice mouth. You got a nice mouth.

Watch your teeth, asshole.

Blondes.

Children. Sixteen could be eighteen to that fucking blob at the door. They want to learn and are so worried about AIDS but give up so easily. Fun would be watching them trying to get to sleep at night: hating themselves. And their bodies, their cocks, their hands and mouths and assholes. And the chance is great that they'll pass it on to some – innocent – victim.

Big brown two-tone dicks that hook. Bellies that get in the way. Cunts who want to play trade.

They are all the same.

The only personality is the wood inbetween. Painted black. Which is what you fuck. And what you're here for.

First it works like this. You trot in so full of lust and stupidity and all you do is feed yourself to the animals. Desperate little doggies who want, simply, a cock in their mouth and cum, sometimes, in their throats.

You look into their little world of videoscreen and locked plywood and watch them tug their hard-ons and pull down at their balls. Bend to check their faces: race, job, style, approach, looks, manners, mistakes, attitude, size. Then you fuck it. The wood with tongue and warm teeth and fucking lousy technique.

    Cumming is cumming. After awhile you piss. You have your shithole lunched out. You get notes. Instructions. Please, sir. Money. Visitors. Friends. Barking dogs and lessons.

    And when you start to learn the meaning of glory holes and easy faggot sex you understand that you have to suck cock. Because that, actually, is what you want.

    There's no such thing as a top or a bottom. There's deluded cartoons and posey safes. There's fags. There's niggers. Cocksuckers. Ugly limp dicks on old men who you can actually watch twitch into Parkinsons'.

    And then you start to measure. You start to make up stories and personalities and meaning. You start to desire and search and worry less and less.

    And you don't like it.

    Eating male is the exact same thing as fucking a cunt. Fucking an asshole is sucking some cunt and fingering some clit. Getting slammed on all fours, your asshole rimmed and rosebudded from a plastic fat slimy dildo and your intestines soaking up someone's puddle of cold cum looks just like your father popping inside of your mother's inhuman bestial slash. With her eyes shut tight just like you.

    He doesn't care anymore.

    But he does it again and again.

    The boy was sitting facing the wrong way when he went into the booth. All ready to finger poke or cock feed, he was surprised a bit by the eye facing the wrong way staring at him through the hole in the wall.

    He bent down to whisper: Fuck off.

But the boy bent down and laid on the cold concrete floor. He put his eye into the hole to see where the boy disappeared to.

The boy huddled on his knees, on the floor, like he was praying to Mecca. The boy was completely naked. His naked boney back and ass cheeks clearly visible in the blue flicker video wash.

The boy dug into his asshole with a backwards hand. He was shoving a dildo in. Further. Out and in again. A dark dildo that was hard to see. Size being important, suddenly, again.

The boy slowly raised back up to see if he was watching and interested. He was. Huddled back down. In and screw; further; in.

Up again to see the reaction, the boy now wants to see a cock. Wants to suck on it. Wants to service. Wants, obviously, to eat cum and drink piss and lick the shit off of fingers he'll dig in only for that meal: nothing else.

But he wants to see more.

The boy bends back in his kneel and displays his soft loafing cock, he grabs his balls and penis in his hand and bunches, tugs and droops. He prays to Mecca again.

Hands back to his ass. His face lays flat on its side facing the showhole and he starts to dig without the tool. He spreads his cheeks far. He moves his head and stares flat down at the floor. The video colors his back but the hole he's playing in is obscured by dark.

The boy is shitting. There in the booth. But he can't see the shit or the squishes, or dirt, just the strain read in his back, hands and face focused hard on the floor.

He starts to rub his pants, his crotch wants some of that messy shithole. Some mouth. Some of

this fucking filth.
   The boy has won and comes up again. Presses his tongue through the wall and wiggles it out. Look for shit. Do you eat your own shit? Do you smell your shit? Cock slides in neat and fills the warmth inside that hole. The boy laps it long and presses his lips all the way to the splinters. Hungry, angry, giving like a mouth slave, a mouth pig, a human male cunt.
   He gets hard and time starts to dull. He pulls out. Soaked. Shit stink cheese. And knows the boy wants something else anyway. He backs away, straightens out, and beats off a little. Shows the boy his sloppy work. Let's him admire the mess he's made: what he wants, he pretends.
   The boy gives him a little yellow post-it note. Carefully printed beforehand in neat faggy pencil.
   FAG WANTS TO SERVICE. TREAT HIM AS YOU WILL.
   HAVE YOU EVER WANTED TO BEAT SOMEONE TO DEATH WITH YOUR BELT? THIS IS YOUR CHANCE.
   DO WHATEVER YOU LIKE.
   Death registers in his head. His cock has lost its girth as he waits and he sizes up the scene.
   Another fag with AIDS. Another death just waiting for time to take him away in sick parts. Another stabbed and bleeding dog for the hot garbage heap.
   He wants to see him in the light now. See the Kaposi's. See the scars. The cancer. Smell the AZT. And feed him his body's wasted dead cum. That is what the boy deserves. What he thinks he needs. Right now.
   Needle marks. Clothing stores that accept

donations only. Old mothers and sisters and candle light parades. This is what smells here. Perfect. The hard-on starts to beat again in his balls and greases up his asshole.

    He turns to the hole and drops his pants to let the boy taste his shit. But then he figures, quickly, that he doesn't want to be naked here. Wants to feed this dying boy loads of human garbage and then, yes, beat him into a crying begging angelic bloody pulp. His boy eyes puffed out red and shut black and blue. His lip three times its usual fag droop size and seeping blood and embedded teeth torn into and out. His nose slashed and broken.

    The belt buckle should be concentrated only on his face. Let him live with a face like frankenstein for the last year or so into his wet hospital bed. Make him blind before the lack of blood cells does. Make him deaf. Knock out every tooth in his lumped and broken skull.

    And leave his prick alone. That point of entry. That lord.

    How helpless can you be. How pinned down and ripped apart till you shriek for the landlord. How much death can you beat. How much can your mind talk your body into deserving?

    He turns back and hitches his pants up. Tucks his cock in and adjusts his balls.

    The boy lowers to Mecca. Probably for the dildo again.

    He keeps the note and opens the door, walks out, and hopes the boy understood he wasn't coming over to his booth.

    I know this fuck-up whose thighs and legs and calves, even his ankles and tops of his feet, are spattered and streaked with long thick deep red

gouges and slices. This beast's particular mania is to be blown while the cocksucker attacks his legs with steel combs and wire brushes. He showed me some scars that came from razors and jackknives. He liked to turn a blow-job into a full on face fuck while he started to feel the sides of his meaty legs getting slashed and scraped and chopped. Motherfuckers jab me and scrape and scratch. When I cum it's so fucking far into their throat I can taste what they ate all week. Some scars were raised red welts that looked fresh, while others seemed to be melding into twisted peach and pink fat flat veins closer to bark than flesh.
     I like to rape their faces. I like to feel them want to get away and hurt me while I attack them. I like my own blood sliding all over myself and the feel of my cumming at the same time.

The inside of that pisshole holds some fascination. The way he pinches the cock head and spreads the hole open between his two fingers. Curls the tip of his tongue into a point and dips it down into the open black pursed space. Discharge. Piss. Nothing.
     Some half nigger fag bends over a wooden plank in a little booth upstairs at the Bijou. The only light comes from a TV monitor showing porn films and the half-caste seems even darker in the buzz and shadow. All you see is his back, half of his face when he turns his head to look at you behind him, and his hands spreading and yanking his ass-cheeks far apart. His asshole is in that black you can't exactly make out just below that quick line of flesh/flicker cathode flash up his boney tail section. When you're inside that asshole, when you feel his weight squeeze against your cock and up into your balls and stomach, you watch only your hands. That

grab his throat and push his neck and head down into his chest and you pump him: cock into fists. He is just this wretched thing you wrapped around your dick. And the noises he makes. The slipping you feel. The rhythm he constantly varies and bucks and blows. And exactly: the way you easily found that little hardly tight hole in the pitch dark.

    I absolutely refuse to wear rubbers. Sometimes I tell them I will and then just leave them off. I absolutely hope to give them AIDS. This specific dysgenic loss didn't even ask. Sucked me hard and needy and turned around and bent spread. Far. Down. Apart. In. And taut. Ridged greased snot flesh. Which, all, certainly, means he's infected.

    In the light he'll look chalky. His mother was black; Jamaican actually. I'm looking for weakness. Sores. I want him to tire quicker and faint and bleed alot more. I didn't feel any shit, I didn't stink when I pulled out, I just pumped out slick and half soft.

    Some other hole, some middle aged faggot on his knees, will lick that smell off of me. Taste this disease's chewed insides and sick. Before that, I have to pull my pants up from my ankles, fasten my belt and button my fly. The nigger gets dressed much more slowly. Measured. He'll want some talk, a hug and a tongue or, much easier, he'll adopt that dogmeat cartoon he likes: used up and lonely and giving and rejected and empty. Fine. I'm looking, as politely as I can, as always, for Kaposi.

    I'll tell you this:

    I've been in that booth before. The very same one. Lots of times. I've been in most of these. Some have just holes in the sides so you can pick the dick you like best of two. Some have only one hole. Some don't have holes. A few have monitors, seats, planks or room enough for more than two.

The last time I was in this booth, I sat on some queen top's neck and shoulders and fed him cock. Faggots watched through the glory holes. He beat himself off while I humped and pumped into his mouth and across his face, my one hand on my cock all over him, the other alternatively a clenched fist left in the air just above his forehead or clamped to the edge of the plank to steady my more violent shoves.

He wanted to be slapped. I wanted to piss. But didn't. He tried to stick his fingers, and his tongue, into my asshole but I was sat too flat and let him know by remaining that way. He didn't want me to cum in his mouth. I didn't. But on his cheek and forehead and into his hair. I was doing most of the work on my dick, keeping it going and bent toward his slobbering gump so he could lick and slurp and pretend he was getting somewhere. He kept his mouth clamped tight and got mad after he peeled himself off the floor of the Bijou's blow-job booth.

I know this cunt liked it. I know he thinks I'm an asshole as well. I know exactly what he jerks off to at home. He wishes he could have taken some of that jism into his throat and across his clenched little teeth.

I've been presented with assholes rather than cocks at the holes. I've been offered cops' mouths and friends' shared erections. I've tasted cock that tasted like my last meal.

I know what a bad blow-job is. I know what makes it lousy: I know what I'm looking for, not what some fucking god has designed for me to find. And a bad blow-job is anything but sloppy self-concern and scraping teeth.

There is a beast that sits in the middle booth at Adult Books on Clark. As you walk to the back, before the stage area where drugged slatterns implode behind glass for dollar tokens, there are two rows of preview booths on either side of the walk. Four booths to a row; three of the booths on the right have open glory holes. The first booth has its glory hole shut with paper and cardboard and tape. It costs a dollar to get in the shop. For browsing. The preview booths take quarters. The video lasts for maybe a minute and there are quite a few channels to choose from, though only a couple will be clear and free of tape wear, static or tracking glitches. Very cheap. And if you're the overly excited type, the shop workers usually don't check to make sure you're feeding the machines.

However, the red light above the entrance to your booth that lets the workers know your screen is on, also alerts cruisers to your presence.

More often than not, there'll be the beast in the middle booth. Something you can stuff your cock into. The beast will be sat, panting and sweating, to take it from either side.

More often than not, this beast will be one specific mistake. A huge fat white bearded and balded blob blubbering over a small wooden stool with his pants bunched down around his ankles, his Y fronts clearly stained and held only half way down his legs. His belly hangs far over his thighs, his penis is only visible when he leans far back to pull at it: to show you he's interested, actually. He is perpetually soft and has the smallest dick ever. Virtually no shaft at all. The tiniest little helmet head and balls that seem sucked up inside his puckered bruised moldy immense girth.

You see this quickly. As you scope. And decide.

He spends the better part of his day here sucking at long cock. He presses his bloated puffed face up against the wall and jabs his short gross stuck Santa Claus tongue at you. He ties up the action for hours; the suburban cocksuckers are defeated by his hogging the middle booth and thus controlling all possibilities. It's get sucked, by him, or nothing and nobody else.

He's learned to suck cock. The way you hate, actually. Professional faggot style with an overwhelming need, abnegating lust pig burn. The inside of his fat face, his deformed and pressured skull, his short bulged winded cheeks and slob tongue are, at once, designed to tell you all of this: Gut fat sucking to give you what he wants. A cock in his head, bobbing up and down, licking the bent forward shaft and housing and brushing the spongy angry head.

Put your balls through.

And you jerk at yourself by slamming up against a wall while he licks and pokes and presses and pops at your hairy sac.

You want me to tell you when I cum?

And he doesn't answer. Fair enough. You have to stare at the wall, you have to consciously imagine: fat fuck, squatting, pulling and pinching at himself, his teeth, his tiny poke, holding and forming and squeezing and flobbing his pigness. You fuck: his entire head bashes up and down more violently on you, never slowing down, he stopped sliding and slurping and staring as he decides this is now the time for you to cum into his hog throat.

You'll draw back smelly. Like his face. And drier than his mouth that gulped directly into his mauled guts.

There is a boy hooker who, a year ago maybe, wouldn't suck your dick. Would only give you a hand-job and figured he was only there to be sucked off.

Fine. Just jerk me off and drop your pants. Let me watch you play with me; you understand.

He hung around outside, mostly, too young and cash obvious to last for long inside where the proprietor used to get nervous easily. He'd want you to take him home, to a motel or for a cup of coffee which meant a nearby alley – which, because of his well known reputation in the neighborhood was a very dangerous and stupid prospect.

He's older now. And just another fag. I think he works at a porno theatre down the block.

And he knows me. And I don't even see his miserable hung white cock and skinny flat stomach while he sucks and eats and asks me to let him know before I'm ready to pop.

I hope to fuck he's dying. I would bet my life on it.

I know it's none of my business but...

What is the correct way to jerk off an old man? So that he'll cum quick and not cause too much trouble: not complain about the money, not try to force your head down to his struggling hard-on, not pull at your nipples through your cheap second hand/second day T-shirt or pull bruises into your balls, thighs or ass.

How to keep him content and stupid and away from the realization of his dog status.

How to just keep the singular focus. The

idea that you're only going to do this and nothing else and the right kind of talk that understands, accepts and just not quite desires. Coddling and sharing and affectionate selflessness are those red flag areas that could just as easily invoke rage and real fucking physical danger. Cash ready placidity. And all the available personality of a clean toilet.

You don't want to be beaten up. You don't want to be raped – which, in this case, is defined by price and chemical disposition. You need to be paid. And you'd like to be able to wipe his cum off the car seat with your hand. Not your mouth or your hair. It's important.

Some of these men – these overfed, fat, desperate, grasping, lazy men – are physically nauseating. Beyond their personalities, beyond their lack of self-control and strength, beyond their comfortable mistakes at hygiene and discipline. The money they don't miss. Beyond the skin color and lube. The grease. Making you sometimes vomit up their taste in the outdoor bathroom of some McDonald's or, worse, between the beer isle and cardboard cookie stand onto the tile floor of some dirty 7/11 knock-off at around 3 a.m.

On a busy Friday night in November, 1995, eight to ten police officers raided the Ram bookstore, arresting four men and charging them with public indecency.

The Ram is only ostensibly a bookstore. Once a patron is buzzed through the front door, he sees to his left, a wall of out-dated and worn gay porn rags and, to his right, videos for sale only. The counter that faces the entrance has a large sign advertising the backroom for $10.00. Scrawled at the bottom of the sign, in big angry black marker, is YES! THAT'S TEN BUCKS! NO IN/OUT

PRIVILEGES!

The video room is large and sprawling and surprisingly clean, having been completely renovated not so long ago. There are small video screens showing porn in various rooms but almost all of the space is taken up by black painted booths, some with glory holes, others with just unlocking doors. There are the ubiquitous red lights everywhere. There is a side room that houses carpeted benches and personal video screens in larger – buddy style – booths.

The next month, the Cook County State's Attorney dropped the charges of public indecency. Andy Knott, a State's Attorney spokesman, was quoted in the *Windy City Times* ("Chicago's Gay And Lesbian News-Weekly") as:

"From a legal perspective, this was not a public place."[1]

There was some pressure put on the mayor's office, by the organized gay community who saw the arrests as harassment, to drop the charges. The Ram's window, which displays only a closed curtain, is painted with the legend: A GAY TREASURE. And the owner of the cocksucking emporium, a vocal member of the community, takes that legend very seriously. He quickly rallied support for his cause while the four arrested men struggled to keep the whole episode as quiet as possible.

Even the uncharged witnesses to the arrests preferred to remain anonymous. The week of the bust, one shadowy individual told the *Windy City Times*:

"The police were kicking in the doors of the booths and shining their flashlights onto people."[2]

Because the cruising is done in a dark but open maze – faggots leaning against the entrance of the tight booths, staring and quiet and sizing and posing and hoping – but the sucking and face fucking and rimming and fagging is done behind the closed doors of the individual booths, what the entire building is created for is not considered public.

The reality, here, however, is that "public" translates to something very specific. Something that has nothing to do with the amount of eyes that could possibly view whatever acts performed at whatever time however easily. "Public" accesses the available, wanting, ready and uncontrolled.

The design of the Ram, like the atmosphere of similar blow-job houses (like, for example, the immense Bijou or the heterosexual oriented mall-like circus of North Avenue Books, recently closed due to "public health" violations) offers absolutely nothing to a public. It has everything to do with access and facilitating needs ripped from damage and brutal confusion. It's all very private. And personal.

Public, here, means natural. And natural includes acceptance, need and a larger sense of unity. And all these words, these convenient and empty words, are mere excuses for an overpowering lust – a useless and mindless search misunderstood as drive – that the patrons of these places can't question let alone fight. Which is why nature, like god and love, make such popular stop-alls. It's hard to argue with a hard cock in your mouth.

And the intensity – the singular heated focus – of this natural drive is exaggerated by the violent pall of AIDS that virtually hisses and howls with every tentative cock stroke and tongue probe. It simply can't be helped. Monkeys hooked up to electric shock centers that massage sex and drug impulses.

There is no such thing as nature.

There is no primitivism that allows for, or defines, the ugly silly little degenerate acts you find yourself behind. The ones you give yourself over to, the kind that mirrors failure, backs up lust or surrenders control and sense.

There is no love. Warmth in safety. Motherly care doesn't exist except as very clear mistakes. Like your father understood when he got the fuck out of there.

Respect is a mark of condescension. Pride is empty advertising and only fleetingly fashionable.

Do you know what a mouth pig is?

Details are important. Reality is on trial. Proof and trust and context are everything.

Mouth pigs are glory hole faggots. Cocksuckers. Made, not born. Male.

Only clowns and misfits forgive. In sex. And only lesbians wrap it around themselves as a protective lifestyle quilt. These beasts that crawl in here looking for healing are looking for religion. They find sex because they're lost and sick with themselves. Which is, more probably, a fine definition for nature.

Which may be exactly what you're looking for.

These seething faggots line the walls of peep shows and movie houses, bathrooms and bushes; all running down checklists inside the corner of their little black burning brains. One list alternates with the other; one is philosophical, the other practical. Both are available. The first is

studied:
> Guilt.
> Self-pity.
> Ego.
> Disgust.
> Revenge.
> Weakness.
> Nature.
> Purity.
> Will.
> Love.
> Lust.

The second list slithers all over them: size, weight, that quick lick that'll produce the exact effect: either in the cock or the mouth. So called seduction. So called cute, romance, taste, acceptance.

It is this last list that is so cutting and perfect. Reality lies only inbetween what one wants and what one will settle for.

I can think of nothing, right now, more attractive than watching some faggot rot away live – half life – from AIDS. I've got memories and I've got photos. I've got a notebook and some videos and all sorts of theories and statistics.

Cotton dry and sore mouths hung off skin stretched over skulls so clear it must hurt just to feel the blood in his brain. Collar bones that jut right out of their neck and shoulders, and straight out of the high shadow black and white photos that some cunt art student was apparently so brave to bring to us. High foreheads and lumps, chemo-hair traces and brittle wisps, dead eyes wishing something could stop hurting this much. Long alien gangly arms made of glass bone. A stupid sick baby smile. With those black burns and blotches and scars and pokes and new holes and leaks. Pinched around the edges and raised and puffed out and cruel. Melted seared skin attached to the underside of those spindly arms and just above the eye and on the ankle and his cheek and all the fuck over his back:

      That someone watched flex and bend against the cock he pushed deeper and deeper into that asshole. Watched that spine curve and buck and take that cock into the space behind waist, penis, thighs and intestines. With skin that sits like rolled soaked paper towels inside his guts that rips slightly and seeps with the virus that the good someone plowing into his insides feeds into the whole family in just one loaded pop and spew.

      A tall thin man that, no doubt, reeked HIV, dropped his long soft cut and taffy cock through your side of the hole. He would suck you off later splashing your sperm fully into his sucking swallowing head and licking your cock head back and around while you got soft on display, you figure, for the faggot seeing through the glory hole on the other side of the AIDS death wall. But now he hops his flaccid cock up and about in your booth by wiggling his ass and twitching his feet on the other side. Suck it, he moans. He coos. And you grab its length and massage its underside and rub the tip of the head: where the piss hole puckers up and open. You slurp at it and engulf it with your mouth, hopefully not letting any of the virus into your bloodstream. Into your head. Suck it, he says again. You pull off and try to force a finger inside that piss hole. You want to tear it open. With a long finger and jam that boned digit all the way inside and down into his faggot body and rip the finger through the stem that you sucked and licked and tasted. You want to razor blade that thing in two and wash in the screams and blood and all before he gets hard this time. Before you pull your head away so that he can cum into the air and not into your blood.

AIDS is everything. You don't have it. And he does. And I'm glad he does. It wouldn't be the whole thing – it wouldn't be anything – without this virus that makes you die so slowly and weakly and paints you with every bad luck mistake and ill-thought and, completely, every weakness that forms every bit of your brain and spinal column. You know; your personality.

The inside of his head felt like every other. Warm, wet, piggish and busy. Annoying when ticklish.

I felt what I did. And what I saw. At least I tried.

My hands around his head, my ass clinching and pumping back and forth into the hard head I cupped hard and held steady. I felt his drooly loving mouth and lips and saw his crewed black hair. I knew his eyes were closed except when he tried to look up at me. Which I discouraged by forcing my fingers tighter into the sides of his hair and ears and pumping faster and meaner.

He had started out like all the other faggots: he licked and slurped and brushed and stared. I felt my cock grow harder and harder from the base of my balls tightening to the tip of my stretching fat head. This happened because I settled into the business at hand and let my ass fuck his face. Like a dog.

I felt his bottom lip mostly. His tongue slapped my cock and balls whenever I'd let him. I worked out my own rhythm by spearing his mouth;

by using his head on my hard cock like a bucket slab of hard dying meat on the fat end of a blunt sticky meatpacker's fist.

I know what cock tastes like: hot. And muscle. And you taste your face and brain as you buzz around some alien appendage – some animal design – that requires you to do that right then. Only.

My penis and sac were clean of the stinging sour piss he had splashed and soaked over his face and hung yawn dripping with those dead closed eye winces and shakes. Aimed at his cock because he leaned back unto his wooden floor and thrust his erection at me, one hand masturbating his thick length, the other positioning his body up behind him. On his knees, his head now at an angle furthest away from my standing legs and pissing cock, he tried to waggle his tongue in the air, at me, as I pissed a steady flow from cock and balls to chest and shoulders back into that faggotty cloying face.

Don't you fucking spit it out. Don't you fucking dare.

Glistening and slippery and formed in my waste, he glommed onto my cock and started to suck. I felt his cheeks draw in and his hand run up my leg and thigh to my balls.

He had told me before he had waited for this. He had blown me before at a glory hole joint. He asked me, after I pulled out of his sweaty smelling face, to, please, cum in his mouth.

I knew to cum in him.

I smacked his head – on his ear, hard. The dog kept sucking harder, both hands pulling and pushing at my thighs and ass and ankles and all over my legs as he growled and tried to jam his face all the way into my body, my cock balancing him, his whole head rending and sucking and chewing.

I yanked his hair. In thin bunches cupped by the insides of my palms, my fingernails scratching and closing tight around his ears into angry mean direction.

When I cum, cunt, I want to see it spray on you. I want you to lick the air and see me deposit my filth onto you.

He resisted, clearly he wanted it directly in his throat. Into his mouth, behind his teeth, flat and warm and thick on his palate. A warm suppurating sensation in my balls, in my ass and through to my cock to my head and throat. I filled that black hole wrapped around my dick, my pig inside his existence, and felt every drop and spurt hit his gump and lips and queer begging face.

It was a mistake being naked.

I wanted to piss on him again.

He started to lick my balls and moved a finger around to my ass, his head followed between my legs and he started to kiss, and lick and dig.

His hand massaged and jostled and hurt, tightly, messy, desperately, my sinking balls and still thickening red cock.

He started to open my asshole with his tongue. By careful continuous prodding and gentle sucking and pushing his entire face up on, in, on top of my ass cheeks and furrowing his nose and lips into my crack and shithole.

I could work out my shit for him.

Into his gut.

I could feel this in my stomach and in my brain and his sick slick face and hard cock below me, masturbating himself, again, while I clenched and eased and dropped my shit into his mouth and face and smeared all over my thighs and butt and back.

I grabbed his cock. Pumped it and slapped it. Pulled it while I tried to shit. He was wrapped all over me, his cock pointing and struggling to get even closer. In his face, on his tongue, into his body; let him eat it out of my bowels and chew it with his dirty teeth and swallow it into his germed bleating withering body.

I turned to see him. I told him to chew. I watched as he slid a clump of slimy bodily brown shit down his chest and stomach into his pubic hair and grease around his hard-on.

I don't want to play games. I don't have to tell you what to do. I wanted to kick a boot up his asshole, I wanted to squash his penis into his solar plexus and wrench it clean and bleeding away from his corpse with a pair of pliers.

I had seen red blotches appear on his chest. He was tired. He had fainted once before, he told me, after being fucked by a huge rubber dildo. He had been tied down and he fell unconscious – everything went bright white – while someone plowed into his gaping ass with a monster flesh pulling fake dick. That person had upped and left. Left him soaked in ill sweat and failing and naked and sex exposed. Alone and wasted into nothing. Dying: maybe not now but definitely.

He had shown me a video when we first got to his apartment. Of him masturbating. The orgasm was a lot more powerful than he thought it would be, he said.

He wanted me to listen to his tapes, he said. He made his own music. He played a noisy clang and drone thing on his boom box while he showed me this video:

The camera pointed at his thighs and waist, as he reclined on the floor, back up half against the wall, his cock getting stiff, his voice nowhere because of the noise in the small apartment. Stroking, feeling, thickening the gray meat package until, later, cum spat out of the tip of his fist as it covered and yanked on the hard belly slapping shaft and purple helmet. His fat balls stretched and flopped while he smeared himself in his own sperm.

I despise the way this faggot looks sucking cock. Eating shit and lapping it and playing in it like it matters: like some plug dead lost zoo ape. Drinking piss and turning his brain off, giving up control.

There is nothing left after that. And its all still a mistake.

This is that intensity – the hard focus – that, you realize later, rings in your ears over any sort of sense or sentient thought. This is all you; all everyone, you think. This is weakness, but acceptable. This is loss, absolutely, damaged. This noise termed sex bangs and screams inside your ears and veils your eyes as you walk – cruise – around yourself through the glory hole booths and partitions. The Puerto Rican faggot who sees you watching a video. While you wait. Walks in front of you, stares down at your crotch and backs into a black on black wood stall. Leaves the door open and drops his hand to his bunched package: which, actually, means he wants to suck you.

Licking his lips. Closing his eyes. Stroking and pulling down on his dick.

His lower lip is disgusting. That stupid lolling

droop – wet and dark red, deeper red in the dark, and the wanting, pleading, devouring eyes that bleed homosexual pure rote.

And: he'll suck on your dick just like every other head faggot will. And: you'll compare it to others that night and your first and last and in your teens and with someone special, good, or not.

The concentration is crushing. It is the tiny truth behind the games and rules and measuring sticks. You let others define you. Your personality is advertising, armor and open shared desperation carefully, wilfully, clumsily masked. As need, as care, as human. As vapid and fake as the idea of respect or love or tribe that would seek and fail to support it.

There is no such thing as preference.

This is how you molest a child:

YOU AIN'T GETTING OUT OF THIS CAR UNTIL YOU SUCK THIS DICK. YOU UNDERSTAND? DO YOU UNDERSTAND THIS SIMPLE RULE? DO YOU WANT TO LEAVE? DO YOU WANT TO GO HOME AND THINK THAT THIS NEVER HAPPENED?

OPEN YOUR FUCKING TINY MOUTH AND PUT YOUR HEAD ON TOP OF THIS NOW.

Slowly take away their options and you'll get what you want, see what you want to see.

And then your decisions get worse and worse, your reasoning is full of mistakes and holes. And all that bad luck. What you thought was vulnerability.

The fag was still into the game. Personal reasons, bad childhood, lonely little loser. I simply asked him for a towel. I decided not to shower – the situation was just this close to reality and the possibility of him recognizing himself could prove very ugly.

I asked him for the video.

Later on, months later, he would give me his notebooks. He filled these Walgreens spiral sale specials with frantic scrawl immediately after returning home after having spent full days cruising and wallowing in glory hole theatres.

Bijou was open 24 hours.

The Ram closed early morning to noon.

He had often spent two full nights in a row – Fridays and Saturdays, especially: day to night to day to night to day again – upstairs at the Bijou. Not sleeping, not eating, hallucinating when the focus wore through or too thick or when the cleaning crews would make everyone move into the downstairs theatre.

I first met him at the Bijou. Later on I saw his name and phone number scratched on a wall there. Later on I would even see him on the street or in record stores.

My favorite thing is this:

I asked him to record a video of him just talking. No sex. This was to be just for me. I told him I liked his notebooks. I told him it was better than having sex with him which, as I told him long before, I didn't care ever to do again.

He gave me a video of him being play tortured by a cartoon leather fag. He never got around to just the talking. He should have just pointed the camera at his face; at those little bumps and zits and marks that I saw whenever I really looked, and talked to the air. His mind would say the right things. The truth. The porn. The reasons and bad decisions. He made excuses and such, but I had a good feeling that it was far too much to ask. I'm sure it just seemed to be too much work, that's all. Or too boring for too long.

Maybe not real enough or physical enough. There had to be more than just him. Alone. Or there had to be action – had to be back on that fat cock.

I remember, now, where my cock was. And my shit and piss when he grins his mouth to talk. I remember seeing that cock jerk and split when he tooled himself between my legs and thinking whether or not as he jammed his face next to the wall that fed him my dick. I remember, above all, how ugly he was and dog drunk and crushed.

I wish I could have made that clearer.

In an open reply to a Joe Murray's letter of November 30, 1995 wherein Mr. Murray took the clientele of The Ram to task for "sex addiction"; Michael Schumann, the manager of The Ram replied:

"If we follow his line of reasoning we see that in his calculations: bookstore sex = anonymous sex = unsafe sex = AIDS = death. This is clearly based on a whole bunch of very faulty assumptions, not the least of which is that all bookstore patrons are gibbering idiots too stupid to look out for their own self-interest. In fact, however, casual sex plays so big a role in the lives of so many gay men in places other than bookstores that one might reasonably believe that it is an aspect of their lives that they do not want to change."
(*Windy City Times*, December 7, 1995)

"Q & A! Q: HOW MANY COCKS CAN A COCKSUCKER SUCK WHEN A COCKSUCKER CAN SUCK COCK? A: 12 (B-I-G THICK DICKS)! About Part 2 of Glory Hole Quartet, Tom says 'Come with me tonight to my own private

"confessional" booth where your hot rugged type of man is shoving his big schlong anonymously through that cum-N-saliva dripping plywood hole to get serviced, worshipped, cleaned up, and shot off!'
    LIP SERVICE, INDEED!
    PIGPEN GLORYHOLE FEAST!
    ALL U CAN EAT!
    GLORYHOLE ACTION the WAY-OUT WAY you lived it! TWELVE (12) BIG COCKS, so commandingly hard, teasing, ramming through the drilled gloryhole, YOU'LL FALL IN LOVE WITH THE PANEL OF PLYWOOD! GREAT COCKWORK! HUGE VEINED COCKS WITH LUSCIOUS SKINNED HEADS TOPPING LONG SHAFTS! TOTALLY TUBULAR! A RAW, BIG DICK WORSHIPPER'S DREAM OF WILD STUD COCK. Real MacWhoppers! All AMERICAN SAUSAGE! Jockstraps, jeans, cockrings. VEINS! JUICE! PRE-LUBE! MULTIPLE CUM SHOTS. All the Olympic Glory of big cock worship at it's RITUAL, PRIMEVAL BEST! Pagans and New Age Male Warriors, come strengthen your manhood! 12 BIG CUT COCKS! 96 rip-snortin' minutes."
(GLORY HOLE QUARTET VOLUME 2; TOM'S CUM CRAZY COCK-SUCKER, Palm Drive Video)

"This is an all oral video featuring our beautiful and BUSTY DE DE. This one is done using the peep show theme. This little 5' blonde loves to suck cock and once you see her in action you will be convinced.
    This video has seven excellent facial and in the mouth cum shots. As we said DE DE loves cum!"

(DE DE'S PEEP SHOW, 60 minutes, Fantasy Video)

This cunt. This fucking beast, this thing that is every female cell on its knees stretched apart from birthing like a back alley plugged and pulled rat, looks at a glory hole cut through flimsy standing press board and mutters, almost imperceptibly, "please let me suck your cock".

You fucked this hole before. Shot cum into it, blind, into its licking mouth and spewed up your insides into its head.

And so you feel the cup in your back and the strain in your thighs and calves as you crouch uncomfortably to slop your cock in the hole and keep it there while you feel: whatever it is rubbing and brushing and flicking and heating along your cock that is blackly lost to you at this time. While you stare at a wall. While you stare at a television screen. This close and blank. And focused and dreaming you're imagining the scene through a dick that may or may not be sloppy wet. Through a dick that isn't yours. Inside some hog's face. A fleshed out wall for a face and a brain. That you fuck, moving your ass cheeks barely back and in their heads again. That you fuck with your fist.

That dead mouth is never female. Unless it's your wife. Or your sister done in a frenzied confused minute. Or a back alley rape where time just won't permit the little porno show you'd prefer.

Women, quite simply, are paid.

This ugly strain of narcissism can give way to a gross misunderstanding of empathy. A mistake that separates gender into two distinct and untenable camps based on similarity rather than difference. Somewhere, there is a special, heavily crowded, brightly lit, hardly safe little quarantine reeking of medication and stale pain with a big fucking red sign on the door: Mouth Pigs.

But this is female trash named whatever. A prostitute. A wretched animal devoid of anything but her most disgusting outward attributes. She is virtually chinless. She even fucking wears glasses. Her blonde hair is crimped and curled in Southern Illinois truck stop lot lizard style and repeats in moppish shakes and jabs the action it hides by bad camera angles.

She barely licks it. Her slurping is fairly noiseless and her workmanship is steady and dedicated and unquestionably indicative of brain death brought on by years of drug and general, easy, body abuse.

How much did she get? And how many cocks in a row spread out over how long an afternoon before she had to return to her job dancing in a peepshow in some backwoods white peeled round red lightbulb adult bookstore. With men in the backroom waiting. With money. With ideas. With a camera and a little more money, today, when you think about it, for even less work.

The first two dicks she pokes through her turgid skull, she pillories herself upon naked. Except, of course, for black high heeled shoes. Her breasts are long and flabby and flattened, watery and jiggery like little clumps of sucked out sand bags refilled with cancerous fiberous loose veins and too much skin. Pink nipples dotted and uneven and hanging towards her belly. Which is in sections because her ugly middle aged pigness attempts to suck it in. Demurely. Pathetically. Uncomfortably.

The lower part of this reptile's white gristled

stomach bulges out from its navel mid-way and cuts and digs into deep winding puckered and pinched stretch scars and cellulite. Her pants must have left those permanent lines that split the fatty deposits that bag over into lumpy sick ant parts.

Her cunt lies below hidden and tucked into more flesh and sparse pubic hair. Her thighs are, too, littered and poked with more cellulite and veiny bruises.

Women are pigs. Toilets. All of them; every single one of them is this drugged-up and raped piece of street forgotten father fucked trash.

Any beast that births. That can birth. That owns the capacity to shit a child slowly through its fatted bleeding cunt. Whore sensitive tits fill with something to feed the bawling needy turd and whose mind becomes soft with tiny little ideas of what love really is, how spirituality really feels and what heaven is whenever you get out of its bed in the stinging hot morning.

This hideous old used cunt puts her clothes on after two blow-jobs. A teddy and long thigh-high stockings slick looking like leather in the right light. Leaves her glasses on throughout. Towards the end she rubs her saggy dugs and pets her cunt through a different outfit: white teddy and lacey satiny panties. She doesn't – is careful not to, in fact, obviously – drag out a breast again or pop her bush. The director, no doubt, told her not to.

The cunt pets her face with one or two sloppy cocks after they shoot inside her hollow head. The cunt lets her bottom lip hang lap dog open so that long white strings of sperm slide slowly out to her bunched up folded full and spongy cancer belly.

She is typical of her age. Desperate and ugly

and aware of her position: worn and hopeless and in need of whatever it has to do, or to be, or to perform, immediately. Only now.

Nothing good can ever come out of a blow-job. Except for the pleasure that might be there in the degradation – the expressed and explicit pained and confused degradation – of the thing wrapped around any hard cock.

This fat cunt works on seven different cocks like a mindless hole, like a washing machine, like an old beaten clanking and burning sloshing and rinsing machine like your mother or sister sagging into what should be some sense of comfort and experience. But here it isn't. Here it is thoughtless. Animal. Nigger. Stupid and weak upon weak; wet instinct as facile but pure reality. Sickening reprobates feeding on each other's seething confusion-cum-anger and wide eyed asking-for-it loss. You move that way and get more of it. Heaped on top of you to drown you slowly, crushing your lungs after your brain and previously masked personality.

You don't want to make these mistakes. You want to enjoy these mistakes. Amateur videos are made for a very small and dedicated, specific, audience. Sold absolutely everywhere.

1. STATES ATTORNEY DECLINES TO PROSECUTE RAM PATRONS, *Windy City Times*, December 7, 1995.

2. FOUR ARRESTED IN LATE NIGHT RAID AT RAM BOOKSTORE, *Windy City Times*, November 16, 1995.

TWO

"Most often, 'soft-core' means pornography that someone thinks is okay; 'hard-core' is pornography that someone thinks is the real stuff, dirty, mean, and at least a little abusive and repulsive. 'Hard-core' has the aura of breaking taboos around it and pornographers use it in advertising as a point of pride."
(PORNOGRAPHY AND CIVIL RIGHTS, Andrea Dworkin & Catharine A. MacKinnon, Organizing Against Pornography, 1988)

"SHE SUPER SLIDES THAT MONSTER WEINER DOWN HER THROAT EVER SO SMOOTHLY, PICKING HAIR OUT OF HER TEETH, CHOMPING WIDE BONERS, AS SHE DRINKS THE FRESH NUT NECTAR DOWN HER THROAT. SHOT THIS IN TWO PARTS THREE WEEKS APART. SHE FIXED HER HAIR BETTER THE SECOND NIGHT."
(THE DOCTOR GETS LAID #3, 90 minutes, AVS LTD.)

"One of my claims to fame is that I knew the dog even before Linda [Lovelace] did."
(THE MAD SATYR pt.1, Jamie Gillis, *Screw*, January 4, 1988)

"In one scene, the dear child is seated in front

of a two-way mirror combing her hair. Unbeknownst to her, but to the horror and amusement of the rest of the cast and crew, I masturbated behind the mirror within an inch of the precious little snot's nose."
(THE MAD SATYR pt.2, Jamie Gillis, *Screw*, January 11, 1988)

"We started as revolutionaries, became filmmakers and ended up as whores."
(THE MAD SATYR pt.3, Jamie Gillis, *Screw*, January 18, 1988)

"No, Jamie isn't crazy, just misunderstood. People expect the worst from him and are surprised to discover he's not the monster they imagined. Sure, sometimes he seems like a sleazy guy, but what the hell is porn all about?"
(RAW TALENT, Jerry Butler, Prometheus Books, 1989)

"'Jamie Gillis is by far the most perverse person I've ever met', Savage admitted with respect."
(SAVAGE LOVER; FETISH PORN STUD RICK SAVAGE, Pearl Chavez, Nugget, 1996)

"Having, himself, taught learning annex classes in the Bay Area and having just completed some other course in film making, Gillis is very enthusiastic about bringing this kind of information to the fans and the adult business wannabes."
(JAMIE GILLIS TO HOST ALL-DAY XXX SEMINAR, *Legal News & Views*, AVN, May 1994)

"So when Gillis announces he's putting on a seminar to teach ordinary citizens how to make saleable adult tapes (though admittedly more of the amateur variety) that's not only news, it's worth attending simply to listen to anecdotes at the master's feet."
(JAMIE GILLIS TEACHES "PORN SHOOTING FOR BEGINNERS" COURSE, *Boneyard*, AVN, September 1994)

"This is a real life documentary style video. It shows Renée Morgan, our female chauffeur, Mondo and myself cruising around San Francisco. We pick up guys and video-tape them doing whatever they want to do with Renée. This is all unrehearsed, real live action. I guarantee it. —Jamie Gillis."
(ON THE PROWL, 65 minutes, Jamie Gillis Video)

"He's At It Again... 'The Prince Of Perv' Jamie Gillis Has Hit The Streets Again In Search Of The Elusive...Exclusive...Ultimate Wet Dream Queen. This Time Ol' Jamie And His Everready Handy-Cam Takes Us On A Steamy...Sweaty Outrageous Limo Ride With A Wild Eurasian Beauty Whose Backseat Antics Is A Zipper Meltdown... Then We Meet A Young Street Honey Whose Back-Alley Gymnastics Will Leave You Breathless... And It's On To The World Famous 'Century Club' Where We Get An Up Close And Very Personal View Of Blonde Super-Star Taylor Wayne... A Girl Who Really Takes Her Fans To Heart... This One Will Really Make Your Hair Stand On End... As Well As Anything Else You've Got Handy. It's The Hottest Pro-Am Ever... And It's A Sin City

Exclusive."
(ON THE PROWL AGAIN, 77 minutes, Sin City Video)

"On a recent trip to Paris, a French producer asked if I'd direct some S/M films for him. We never actually closed the deal – but I did shoot these casting sessions. The first two girls I saw were brand new to S/M – after putting them through their first spankings, they both decided they wanted to try being in charge.
    The new-born dominants seem to have the most fun when one sits her beautiful, young ass on my face while the other whips my crotch with a belt.
    The third girl is well known in Paris as a bitch with her very own torture chamber. She likes to treat men like dogs – literally – and has me barking to her heart's content."
(JAMIE'S FRENCH DEBUTANTES, 60 minutes, Dungeon Video International)

"1. Jamie delights in handling bad girls with a sound spanking. Tiki, a tall blonde with big tits, confesses, while being spanked, that she had sex with her boyfriend's best friend. Jamie uses his hand, mini whip and belt as he puts Tiki in unusual positions and turns her tender ass bright red.
2. Jo Jo has a beautiful bottom, nipple rings on both nipples and an attitude. Jamie once again uses his large, firm hand and mini whip. Jo Jo admits that she has been spanked before. Jamie has her sit up in his lap, hugging Jo Jo as he punishes her trembling, glowing buttocks."
(MORE BAD GIRL HANDLING, 60 minutes,

RedBoard Video)

"Three different segments on this video & while not as nasty as the WALKING TOILET BOWL videos, it still delivers Jamie's unique style of perversion & the girls are cute! They shit, blow enemas, shit their pants ...Jamie smears shit everywhere and jerks off in the filth!"
(JAMIE'S POTTY GIRLS, 110 MINUTES)

This had to be explained to her.

  For every cum shot you take in the face, I'll give you an extra five dollars. This is dangerous on my part. Quite generous. Aside from the fee already discussed and agreed upon – a flat fee that is yours no matter what, as long as you let as many men as I let in here fuck whatever hole of yours they like – the five bucks per shot is extra; and only depends on your taking it in the face.

  That is: if some sweaty nigger hogs himself out of your cunt, having brought himself to the brink of climax by banging away inside of you for however long it took, then, quickly, juts his body up to your head and masturbates himself to cum onto your face, that's extra money for you. Same is true for the men you'll be letting fuck your ass and fists. Obviously it's true for those who'll take your mouth first and foremost.

  None of these men will hurt you. There'll be just over twenty of them. All naked. At times there'll be another girl around to help you and them. All combinations are possible.

  I want to encourage you to suck the men off using your mouth like a jackhammer, use your tongue and your hands. You'll have to be energetic, don't get tired out. With so many men all looking for the next open hole, chance or shot, the quicker they can be brought off, the better.

Lick up their cum. Chances are great, in your favor, that you can't get AIDS from cum inside of your mouth. Anyways, you don't have to swallow. Let the men beat off in your face – they'll push their hard-ons into your mouth and cheeks, rub them over your nose and eyes and hair – while you extend and dart your tongue out and slurp up at the tips of their dicks. Gobble at their balls. This will help them cum faster and it's extra money for you to let them ejaculate all over your tongue and, if you prefer, your closed tight mouth. Even on your nice white teeth which you can keep clenched if you're worried, or if you just maybe like it that way best. The men will aim at your mouth.

Sweat is fine. Towels will be handy. You'll be drenched in their sweat as well as your own. Your hair will be drenched and lay flat wet against your head and back, stringy and hot and uncomfortable. Your nose will dot and drip water.

Don't wipe off their cum. Except if it hits you in the eye. If, for example, you're laying flat on your back and someone jerks off onto your aahing tongue and face and explodes all over your chin, neck, cheek and lips – let the sperm stay where it hits and ooze into the mess of other men's jism that surrounds it. Alot of big wads collecting on your face and tits and whatever is exactly what we want. Our audience like that idea; like that look, so keep that in mind. Let it splash and stick.

It'll be over soon enough. The more cum shots you take in the face – and the men know that's where we want them – the better for you as you'll have all that extra cash when we're done. Some men will cum on your belly or your back after fucking your cunt or asshole and that's fine. Let them. Most will want your pretty face.

Use your hands. It helps the men stay excited while they're waiting for a hole to free up.

Cocks that enter your vagina and anus will have on condoms. We encourage the men to take the condoms off when they're just about to cum and to cum outside of your body, obviously. This will all be filmed. The condoms, if the men cum inside your cunt, or asshole, or even in his hand while still wrapped, will probably be emptied out onto your tits or ass or, preferably, into your mouth. Stick your tongue out and hang your head back and let him squeeze the condom flat out above your wide open mouth. Open real wide and really push out that tongue. The open end of the condom will be pinched above your face, then released. He'll press his fingers down the hanging rubber to let every drop of cum slide out and into your mouth. Wait till he shakes out the last drop. Except if you're choking just a little, then tilt your head the right way and swallow. Then open up again to collect whatever may be left. If you can, let the cum lay on your tongue for the camera to go in for a close-up or at least, to make sure you caught it. Also, if you're really still worried, to let the air kill the HIV virus should it be present. Which I'm sure it isn't. And anyways, the spermicide in the condom would have killed anything so really you just can't worry about it. When you pull your tongue back into your mouth, swallow. Or push out the cum and spit from your mouth with your tongue and let it drool down your chin and neck. That will be worth the same extra five dollars.

Obviously.

    Sitting, naked waist and legs, her armless t-shirt bunched up around her neck to display what little tits perk up, she spreads far apart to further access some moron lapping up inside her sopping wet man after man after man plugged and spewed on cunt. The jerk squats himself down between her gangly legs and aching ankles with his balding head pointed down at the mess. She is flanked, plopped on a schoolroom brown metal folding chair, by two men both jutting half-hard-ons glistening with smelly sweat and her spit. Her head – being the exact correct height for such an act – pivots between the two meats and licks and sucks and jaws at the outsized genitalia, stomaching their nigger stinks and warm hygiene tastes inside her face and memory. Her hands drop to a sac of big balls and back up to the fattening cock as she faces each in turn. She makes an uncomfortable effort to jerk the cock her mouth ignores for a minute or two but usually decides that her coordination works best on a single cock. Both men will eventually use their own hands – their own rhythms and friendly masturbation technique to all but jack off into her face as her tongue lolls and wipes around the spearing and retreating cock head pissholes – and then push their cumming weight further into her mouth as she tries to keep her lips and teeth closed so the cum'll collect on her face and spill down her little perfect tits and thin belly and that cunt lapping middle aged head.

    Men who watch the action, pulling themselves off while they stare, will zombie over to her seat and shove their cocks into her face, rudely, as soon as they think they can't take it anymore. The niggers in the round seem especially pushy.

They are also less likely to settle for a cum generated only by their own fists and eyes.

Lay down, the bulky camera man recording the circus will instruct every now and again. Cum shot, cum shot, he'll bark if motioned by one of the minion and the flesh slapped nest around the beast will open up to allow for the crowning home favorite angle. With one camera, rarely but occasionally two if lucky and the money's there for that and a nicer hotel room, the action is always focused on the whore. Men sit and stand, naked and cold and preoccupied, pulling their cocks, sipping juice or beer just outside of the camera's range or interest. The center becomes her dugs and mouth, her burping cunt and slackened asshole, close-ups of machinery penetration while the sound picks up the guffaws, idle conversations and dog-pound encouragement from those milling about just behind and beyond the fucking and sucking and accepting.

Give it to me. Give it to me. Give me another. I want more cum. Give me another cock. The blank rag will bleat as she worries about the sperm being wasted on areas other than her paid face. She makes it sound like sex talk. And if it helps the conditioned response of porno hounds and worthless niggers cum quicker so much the better. But its intention is capitalist and efficient. Give it to me. C'mon give it to me. C'mon who's next. Baby, baby, baby.

I will never ever do this again.

Sold. What number was that? What number am I up to?

Let it come down. Let it fall. Let it wash all over you. Let it soak in.

It's not the buyer. It's not the market. It's

not that any of it exists out there tenuously in your spindly hard nailed grasp all the time, every day. It's not the cruelty or the lessons to be learned, or the truth in fact.

It's the seller.

The dogs at the door, begging to be let in. And fed. And the bath that they don't realize is good for them. All the rats crowded around and chewing into each other's corpulent splotchy short mat fur meat with their pin prick razor teeth snaps, dig and retracts. The ones that are killed so easily with just a slim wood stickball bat to the back of their brittle twig bendable spines and walnut sized heads. You pick them up dead, avoid the far too small spots of raw exposed red blood scratches and tiny bobble eyes, hold it's dime bag weight by it's ribbed worm fat tail and drop it in the dumpster.

You can easily hold a cat in the air, away far from your body, arms outstretched and stiff as your hands squeeze into it's soft boned neck. The cat will scream and mewl guttural and angry like a choking baby and thrash as wildly as it can. Small shit will drop from its shaved ass and piss will fly in short streams and misses every which way around. Or you can keep its head – its baseball sized head where you can feel its thin skull and quaking brain through the crewed fur and bumps and shut closed tight little kitty eyes – as you rub the clenched head about in a puddle of polyurethane or whatever those turpentine based chemicals are that are so easily available. Watch it fall apart and writhe and struggle and stroke side twitch and choke cold coughs and expire in sliding slow wheezes and spasms long after the poison has made it all but near dead. Don't let it drown.

There's the Id. And the Ego. There's the

young girl finally come unchained. It's all very simple to sell.

The emphasis is all on the one under the pile of pigs at the trough.

Paid in full. Hardly. None of these decisions are easy unless you're down that far already. Right, honey? Then it's just a question of who's going to pay. The amount is important in the negotiating, right? You don't want to be taken advantage of. As long as you're there now. You want as much as possible. You want what you're worth. Or what the act is worth. Considering the time and the market and what that motherfucker will make off of it. He can afford it.

But the truth is that the money isn't really worth arguing over. Because she'll do it. It's a question of degrees, not price. The decision has already been reached. The money is whatever she can be convinced of – of what details she'll retain as to what the men are getting, the rent of the room and the rapidly disintegrating hot Florida mattress on the floor and all the gear.

Beer – not too much – coke, orange juice, poppers, lube and pizza in the kitchenette.

I don't believe you were made for this. I don't believe you don't deserve an upgrade, another shot. Something much better. But I don't see that you have somewhere else better to be just now either. Or an idea that can be better than the single opportunity open to you at just this minute.

So, fine, it's just your hand.

Give me some help here.

He pulls his cock out of his pants and works it up at you. He watches you look down at the exposed flesh, worrying up your next sentence, trying to remember the best route and safest bet.

    The make-up you bathed in. The pants you bought. The fucking string hanging out of your ass as you slip down your panties whenever. The alcohol stain and swallow and the mirror you glance into as you pass. The TV show you decide not to watch, the drug you decide isn't for now but later or maybe not at all. This is all you are everyday. Those quick little minutes better than the long ones. All steady, if possible, all burnt into one tiny train of inevitability.

    The blouse that looks best. Cutting off the end of that tampon or thinking about using it as an all-around excuse. The high heels that pinch your corns and make your calves hard as bricks. The way you jog and skip so your butt cheeks don't look too mushy. The way you stare before you're paid and then after. Your tummy bulge and the muscles that can suck in or relax depending on the time of night. That crick in your back. That taste and memory. That very necessary shot of labelless bourbon or only slightly used flannel sheets.

    Give me a hand.
    Rub the balls.
    That's good, that's good, like that.
    I'll give you an extra ten to just look at your tits. Just pull your top up. I want to look, not touch. I can do it myself.

    Short stubby fingers that reach to tit-fuck you. Miss: Can you please stick your breasts together. As he flops and waddles his pasty heavy male all over your vulnerability worrying and firing beneath mouthwash, a little LSD to make you giggle and every ounce, every year of dysgenic stall all clean and molded just for this.

    Some asshole sits on the subway bench across from you. He's still wearing his shades, looking like a posey pratt, as if he's not staring at you. Checking out what you have to offer; he figures. Your tits, the way you cross your legs, where you avoid looking, your just washed hair and accessories. This pathetic moron thinks to himself that you were made for him. He figures just watching will be enough; just this little bit. He makes the same mistake all these doggies do: he imagines that all mouths are made for blow-jobs. All cunts are the same. All holes just waiting to be filled by him. And his lonely little train dreams are all he'll get. You know this. And laugh: even money couldn't buy what he thinks he wants, though you'd pretend to sell it to him just like anyone else.

    It's only cum.
    It doesn't stain.
    It wipes off forever.
    That's how cheap you are. How cheap you come. What you have to offer and for how much.
    That slide down here was fast. Now, it seems, everything up until this point was fast. But let's not fool ourselves. This is all easy.
    Your life is very easy.
    Tell them what you can remember of what they want to hear.
    Lie about your hard choices: Dad beat Mom. Dad didn't like your older boyfriend. Dad liked certain parts of your anatomy better than certain aspects of your soul, heart and innocence.
    Your brain runs over real choice: the attention your breasts got when you entered the eighth grade. You didn't have a chance to even develop a personality. Those big tits got you what you wanted and you cleverly mapped out a life to follow. Those nigger like lips helped seal the deal.
    Somewhere a mother is just all fucked up

over her morning coffee. Missing its baby. Its ghost pain. Its hole in the heart. This mother remembers and, alternatively, looks for clues and avoids them. Her room. Driving by her high school. Phone calls late at night and none at all for months. Reports. Friends, shopping, smiles of surprise and quietly fed wonder. Lies. Money. Ego. Your fucking wish list.

And a little uncaring titted troll walks the streets of wherever her bad luck flung it to. She is addicted to whatever drug that allows her some personality. And she sucks nigger dick for it. And she sucks white and hispanic dick for money for the nigger.

She doesn't imagine that she is haunting her mother's friendship sleep time. The beast now only knows crack. But, to her credit, there was a time when she knew that her mother only used the idea of a child as the reason for having one. She never really mattered. She never really existed. And she actually proves that now. She and her mother both know she is correct.

How does one explain the fact that one can derive pleasure from the pain of others if that pain is merely born of confusion? Her stupidity forms and protects her. She is a common enough liar. Nothing special.

God allows the others to serve. That little blonde haired rat that attaches its pre-teen lips to the end of its father's hot cock believes in what it has to. It doesn't know what to think. It doesn't have the capacity. It isn't lost as much as it never mattered enough to count. The head count, the line count, passed it by. Mores the pity.

Some skank rotund nigger in a leopard skin t-shirt yanked down the low collar and flopped out a brown tit for me. This was on Halsted Street near the Addison police station so the exposed breast was an absolute necessity. If I would want to see it again, say, like when she jerked me off or blew me, it would have to be figured into her dirt cheap street price. This was just a quick black oily nigger nipple to prove her whoredom. I drove my car up past her and turned around in a parking lot. As I waited to pull out of the lot and head back to the street pig, another black beast ran up to the passenger side and yanked the handle. It wasn't locked. A mistake I wouldn't make again. And this skinny nigger splashed herself right down next to me.

Don't worry. You want to have some fun?

I figured as long as it's not a cop. I wanted a street prostitute. I didn't care if it had big tits like the animal on side show or little hidden ones like the sweaty frantic loss gargling beside me.

You wanna play? You wanna fuck, you wanna real nice fuck?

She told me where to go. I already knew. And then started in on price and my tastes. Which were simple enough. I only had ten dollars and I only wanted a blow-job.

She rubbed my cock through my jeans and asked me if I was clean, which was a first for both. The rest had always been very quiet and hardly excited or interested enough to grope – especially, it follows, for ten fucking dollars.

I assured her I was clean and let her know I was surprised by the question. She blew her cover by launching into stuttered lies:

She usually works around the Gold Coast area. She doesn't work the streets too often, gets most of her traffic in the bars around there. But, see, she was arrested just the other night and decided she would work around here for awhile til the heat cooled down. Then she pointed to a paperback book she was carrying and her small purse and said she had these with her to really come off legit.

She liked to pretend that she was waiting for the bus there. She said.

It wasn't until later, driving home, that I put all this together. The blow-job she gave me was certainly unlike any other I'd ever had. Especially from a hooker. Especially from a street pig such as the kind available in that neighborhood at that time of night. She sucked in on my balls and licked my thighs and rubbed my cock with her tits. She flicked and kissed the head of my hard-on. In the middle of working, she asked me if I liked to fuck. I, of course, told her I didn't have enough money. But she didn't mind: she asked again. Do you like to fuck. She started to shimmy out of her pants and kept her nigger lips and rushing angry tongue washing all over my hard dick. I could see her wirey pubic hair just a little in the dark in the car and I saw more of her ass as she shifted it up to peel down her pants and panties. I told her to forget it. That I was going to cum. But she kept wiggling and sucking at the same time. I think she was patting and pulling herself. Fingering and running her nails through that brillo nest of kept sweat and yeast. Trying to convince me.

I came in her mouth and she backed off but, unlike every pig cunt face that I ever fucked for money before, she kept at it. She kissed and licked around where the cum may or may not have slid and cooed and kept stroking me. Sucked and popped at my balls again.

I thanked her. And pushed her nappy head

away from my now very sensitive still stretched cock, wet and sticky and exposed. She started to get hold of herself and then asked me: full face to face. Was it her looks that made me cum so quick or was it just 'cause I ain't had any in a long time. Or maybe it was her technique. Her tongue and mouth. I told her I was married, though I wasn't, and yes, it was a very nice blow-job.

She was waiting at that bus stop.

That book was some little thing she brought with her to read while the dollar bus took her back home to wherever south she lived. The far south side of Chicago is all ghetto. But I figure this one had to have a real job. She saw the hookers around. She knew where they took their tricks. Maybe she worked on the north side and knew what she wanted to try out one night.

Prostituting her mouth and empty head was what she was drawn to. And, I think, made for. She saw it there all over. And, perhaps, when she saw me pull into the parking lot to pick up the titted beast I had just passed, she figured she'd give the game a quick reckless try.

It couldn't have been money.
It didn't seem like her life.
Until now.

It was virtually the only option open to her. What with that mouth. Like having big tits on a teenager. And like working all the excuses out later. Like pornography.

Accepting is different from settling. And forgiveness and healing and fantasy and empowerment don't even enter into it.

Her mother worked so hard to keep her out of the drugs and gangs and wasted mind of the ghetto. And she and her god are so proud now. It all worked out so well. Just a little dalliance. And the future is still wide open.

You have to reach down so far into these pigs' mouths to get any sense of separation. Any effort on your part will hardly be rewarded. Desperate stereotypes who've given up, who've lost, who didn't have a chance or didn't want one.

The bruises they sport and don't care about hiding is the only thing that gives them some degree of personality. What someone did to them is what makes them special, makes them tolerable. In fact, worthwhile. Human.

The little pig raped by whoever, whatever the relation, however violent the surprise. However unfair the attack. However brutal the trauma, however real the life seems packaged. The little holes sold into bigger ones. The mouths that no longer just eat and bark. The bodies that no longer just shit but accept pain and cancer under the idea of necessity. Of desire. Of cause and effect. Of malleability. Of what's left to sell.

The older woman who now looks into a mirror and wonders. Constructs a plan on how to accurately paint up the toilet seat that stares back at her.

I've got an extra five dollars for the best tattoo. The boys that have ones that say "NO CURE" and the girls that say "SIXTEEN YEARS OLD" are particular favorites.

They'll crowd around you. While you lay down. And while you sit up. They'll slump into couches and onto folding chairs and the sides of lamp tables and it'll be your job to go to each one in a row, sucking them off and stroking them as they recline back, their pants crumpled down around their ankles. As if they're masturbating in front of their TVs alone at home.

They'll collect in a circle. Standing. You on your knees. Turn your head, now go in order. Nigger, nigger, nigger, white and thin, yet another nigger. About ten all closing in on you, soft meaty thick spit wet and slimy cocks selected for their size being worked on by their own hands as you move to the next, then the next, then the next, tasting your own mouth now instead of their individual cocks.

Her cunt is cramped with a purply dick having replaced some stranger's two knotty fingers. Her breasts – lubed with nothing but sweat so as not to scratch – are being squeezed and flopped on one side by a man kneeling next to her as he pulls on his very hard cock waiting for a chance to stuff up any part of her; the other side of flabby dug is being manhandled by the faceless dolt who slips his flaccid cock into and back out of her mouth for useless licks and slurps. She switches his cock with another, this man kneeling far too close to the tit grabber cock handler. Two of the men will cum about the same time – the ones sharing her mouth – and shoot their wads directly down into her wide open gullet gaping throat.

They'll move her over, bend her back so her asshole points slightly up. Some geek will shimmy underneath her and slip his hard-on into her slimy cunt as she lies baby oil flat on top of him. Another will squat behind and above the coupling and slowly fit his forced down uncomfortably cock into her shithole. The two men will eventually settle into a rhythm that uses her body as a heavy dead piece of masticated holed out beef. All the while she'll turn her head, under all this bulk if not activity, arch her back so that'll hurt certainly the next day and suck on another pair of head switching beating cocks. Her hands have to steady and support her fucking sandwiched body so any more hand-jobs or masturbating help is out of the question. The background is blurry with men watching and pumping themselves. Or leaning and talking and laughing and drawing the director to the action he might miss by obsessing on the wrong filled hole.

Her stunted eyes. Her rabbit tongue. Her red puffed and oily pimples and lack of make-up. Her lumpy tits. Her fatty unhealthy ass cheeks. Her little tummy and female rolls. The way her eyes automatically close as the first spurt of cum jettisons from any pisshole directed straight at her face.

The stupid words she thinks and drools out of someone else's mouth in all that fog and buzz.

The instructions that she takes. That make it through.

The way she waits til each fuck finishes before moving again, before even thinking.

"Our sexy lady is staying over a friend's house but falls asleep. When she awakens she finds the house full of the bride's father's friends and the Groom's friends. She seduces the bride's father into joining the party. They watch together at what happens. She watches a girl do a striptease and as she gets more excited she thinks she can do better. She is invited to join the crowd. As the show continues she begins her own show by showing off her legs and sexy body in a dress that is too tight and too short. What happens next is a sex orgy beyond belief as she takes on more than 20 guys again and again. She sucks them all

then goes from cock to cock being fucked. This girl just loves to have a guy cum and she makes them cum more than once till she takes more than 29 cum shots herself in a cum bath explosion. When the party is over the girl decides to leave but some late arriving friends feel left out. These guys want something special. The girl decides to give it her all even when she finds out they all want to fuck her in the ass. She does her best taking one cock after another in her ass but first they shove a dildo up her ass and she masturbates with it. This video set has more action and more wet shots than any other videos we ever made available with one lady."
(GANG BANG #17 – THE BACHELOR PARTY PART #1, 100 minutes, A&B Video)

"Tanya cums home to find her boyfriend has some new Gang Bang videos from A&B. She gets off reading the descriptions and winds up in her dreams seeing herself being Gang Banged and taking a Cum Bath. First she finds herself in a circle of guys who each sits on a stool while she sucks them off she goes from fantasy to fantasy as cock after cock goes into her mouth and pussy. Cum shoots out on her face and tits again she finds herself surrounded by more guys as cum oozes all over her till she ends up taking 23 CUM SHOTS til she is bathing in cum from cocks and condoms she doesn't miss a drop of her Hot Wet Sticky Candy."
(GANG BANG #44 – TANYA EATS IT ALL, 100 minutes, A&B Video)

"This lady loves fucking and loves cum. First she entertains a group of men in a wild fucking orgy that ends with them all giving her face a cum bath. Then she tells them she wants to eat their cum and brings out a dish. They again fuck her but end cumming on the dish. When they have all spent their last load she takes the dish and eats their hot cum licking it up into her wet mouth."
(GANG BANG #70 – CUM EATER, 90 minutes, A&B Video)

It's a heavy uncircumcised cock. The thin foreskin covers about three quarters of the long pink head even when hard. There's lipstick – cocksucker red – all over the wet pisshole and tip. He yanks it out of a mouth doing female jack hammer hard work. Cradles his meat – his cock and his balls – with one free hand and points the straight out hard-on downwards with a painful but simple stroke. Not far. As he's standing, she's kneeling, and he's just a little back bent to fit himself rhythmically inside her face. As he readies to climax, he tends to straighten up if barely arch slightly backwards in fake porno ecstasy style.

His cum spits out of his cock in thick fluid pumps. Aimed at her mouth, primarily; his ejaculate spills all over her face. He tends to paint the face when he cums: rubbing and jerking and almost imperceptibly stopping as each spasm produces another thick white splash. Her head has been hung back to catch his cum. Like an ashtray. Like all the rest.

The camera affixed to his other hand and hooked to his eye records all the action cock heavy.

He directs his head, the audience, down and captures the frame as he has done in countless video sales: the head as receptacle. As paid, again and again with as little deviation from this very precise act and response. This woman's body is just a brief stop in a large number of cunts – mouths, vaginas, assholes, personalities – all available to perform this very important, very specific, very rigid and archetypal tableau.

There are other cameras and camera men. Often enough. A bigger budget and greater distribution, professional marketing and above-ground adult video industry sanction allows for, and requires, thinly scripted smiling scenes with self-conscious over-acting designed to collapse just as soon as the sex begins. Which is just as soon as it can. But the focus remains constant. The market divined, settled and mined.

It is objectifying. It is tedious. It is all probably about money, now, after twenty or so different editions. It has always been about money.

Each and every girl displays the same face when the close up money shot is finally delivered: Resolute drudgery.

The bright eyes, the sultry twists of mouth and tongue, the studied and professional hands and stomach shimmies, the deadened dog slurps and clit bobbing needling self-absorption all finish as gilded sales copy as transparent as grade school bathroom excuses. As is perfectly understood.

"Rodney's smutty want ad reads, 'Video Producer seeks Pretty Faces to Cum On'. Brand new girls are responding to this ad. And they're Nasty, the kind of girls who want their tasty butts spanked before they drink cum!"[1]

Buzz words are less relative in the

underground. The honesty can be claustrophobic. The smaller and smaller audience's interest so precise that the relationship between faceless market and corporate marketeer virtually degenerates into more direct, though no less cliched, john to pimp. Typical ad copy is rendered capricious and insulting as the words, rather than thinly masking comfortable and new-age safe triggers, must now display a shared sense of interest, if not a common responsibility. The pimp's part becomes that of an active participant with an egalitarian dedication to exploration. The rutting drive steeped in coddling and acceptance. The language is precise and obsessive. The concern is recidivist.

Fuck the games. Get rid of the play acting. Let the real thing be sold rather than sipped through even easily deconstructed legalities and unnecessary, fantastic pleasure center guards. Explode the parameters and reduce the false self-denial into simple warts-n-all prurience.

And best of all: it can be done without the girls knowing it.

How do you rape someone that's allowed it? As in the idea of putting a micro-camera in some suburban ladies' room and filming all the heavy winter jacketed fat asses who march in to relieve their lazy selves one after another. Fat cellulite beasts and bladders who allow themselves a quick personal moment away from hiding their pig bodies and sink into their bloated hideous lumpen humanity. If you're lucky, once in a great while, one beast may wipe the wrong way up or maybe clean the toilet seat psychotically before planting her toxic rotting filthy holes down to expel all that ugly pressure inside.

None of these cunts seem to get it. The fact that on the other end of the dick they're sucking at is a camera, doesn't seem to mean anything as nearly important as the money politely slapped to the yeasty insides of their puffy young vaginas, dreams, youth or needle pricks. And that, most important for the audience, the camera here records anything but the sex they think they're selling. Or giving up. Or getting by. So easily, so cheaply.

Let's make it clear. Let's make it personal. Let's carve a new niche in the market.

The whores in any low rent district, dangerous at all times save for a perspicacious adult understanding between thieves, junkies and careful pimps and cops.

The nigger paid to parade her fatty motherly jugs around on the street like the whores you passed by all those times? See the flashing series by Alchemy Productions. Especially *Flashblack* (S10).

Something more direct, see Randy Detroit who fucks ugly black trollops of the kind lined up on street corners in Chicago selling cheap for liquor outside 7/11's and willing, forced, to sell up for a six pack alley way blow-job often enough:

The pregnant skinny titless toothless crack whore he fucks in *The Doctor Gets Laid #3* is full of the same promise you avoid daily in welfare lines spilled out onto the streets and half-minute newsblurps of shit black babies being crib shook or dropped and sold to death.

The fat monster he slides his thick shaved peach white cock into and out of, effortlessly, in *The Hookers Who Loved Me* just lays there blubbering and bored while he pounds away as deep as he can get inside that dark oily stretched and pinched and rolled and huge fat mounds of nigger cunt meat and belly. She zones and stares off blank while he jerks himself off over the flopped indolence and shoots puddling white cum all over the black lard whale of hair, lips, pits and stink. She acts like any paid hooker living inside any cheap hot box apartment would. Paid for her slash. A little extra this time – cause of the camera, the money shot, the time it takes to set it all up for posterity.

A little whisper in its afro haired ear would be nice: Do you have any idea what is being sold here?

But unnecessary.

What part of the woman gets raped exactly? What part of the community?

Because: I'm not worried about being raped. I can't possibly relate. When I look outside, after I've locked my front door and walked down the three flights of stairs inside my apartment building's dinginess, I don't see the potential danger. The heavy handed mexicans, the barking animal niggers, the alcohol crazed white bums don't mean quite the same threat.

The stairs are long and winding with slight dark pockets at the best of day. At night, when I've returned home to find the hallway light burned out, my sense of fear can't be even close to what the women in the building, in the exact same situation, must feel.

Because, apparently, it's just that much worse. And worth protecting all the more.

Really, it must be terrible.

And always just this close; around the corner and dragged in the alley or the seats of any car, or in the hallway, in the pitch with a blood slid skull cracked pipe knocked out half dying and leaving the vagina and anus slack lifeless and accessed easily.

Prove to me that you're more than meat.

Because I don't want her to be all women. I'm trying to make this personal. Between me and her – the fear she felt being weaker naturally and vulnerable and still making that decision to walk up all those stairs trying to feel her way up the side rail. The extra drink she shouldn't have had since she was driving. The slightly larger rent she should have agreed to in a little better neighborhood. The size of her femalia: her tits, lips and the color and feel and selection of her underwear. The condom in her purse and the money shoved into her pants pocket. How long I had to wait for her in particular or someone just like her or anyone with the hardly correct equipment. Her bad luck. Her decision to follow instructions or her saying all the wrong things. The what watching her bleed does to me. The size of the stretch and cut in her flesh and the bottle in hand.

Now: would explaining your intentions to them be the same as rape. Or is the rape part just watching the playback later – for reasons they don't understand or don't even fucking care about. Is it the cameraman's purchase power so blithely lorded over the uneducated but just mildly desperate lapping face. Is it the sale of the tape or the purchase or the relationship formed within a patriarchal buyer's market. Is the rape in taking more than what the whore offered or was previously willing to sell? Is the rape getting it all for so cheap a price? Or that it's all packaged up so easily and immediately, so degraded and low a position so readily accepted, convinced and so inhumanly taken advantage of.

An insult so thin. And sold cheaper.

Forty bucks buys alot of that stuff out on that street.

Say: I'm a good nigger.

"I'm a good nigger" she lets whisper between licks of his hairy heavy sac.

Come up and get some dick.

Lick don't suck.

She acts like a monkey when he tells her to, before the bartering for more cash begins, because it's easy enough for her little black self to do in the price already reached. The blackened rotten banana she waves around and the ape grunts she mimics, the flies she pretends to pick and scratch, don't look and sound all that wrong outside of a crowd.

Jamie Gillis keeps his camcorder tight to his eye and looks down on the nigger whore he pays to eat some of his shit. She twists around and argues with him from inside his half clean but dry crowded bathtub. He offers her an extra five dollars for putting his turd in her bright white toothed black lipped mouth and ups the amount incrementally for chew then swallow. Let me see it.

Vomiting is ok. As long as we can see it.

The price was for shitting on her chest. And we'll see what happens.

Honesty is easy to come by when the situation is as uncomplicated as this. This tight and specific. The price the viewer pays to watch directly supports the action. The implications are personal and pure, the complicity salient.

The trappings and boxes and marketing and ecumenical excuses are all unnecessary legalities under which the truth denies itself and hopes to stop just short of undue influence suits and perfectly unavailable here. You're no longer paying for the advertising. Or the safety. Silicone tits, lip gloss, mascara and high heels, words like sex negativity, empowerment, catharsis and soulless no longer mean what some fat retard lawyer says they do.

These acts are illegal.

These bodies, fucking right, are exploited.

Definitions are made flesh. Words become connections.

David, the cameraman in the *Brown Bomber* series records his dealings with bottom scale street hookers around Los Angeles. He offers to pay them to shit into bowls and onto plates. He films it all – and as he usually has to wait a great deal of time for even the littlest of "nuggets", Dave's constant questioning and the hookers' withered answers and bodies and brains are what's really for sale. Their unembarrassed dirt squeezed and pressed out of unresponding used and drugged muscle functions is the perfect conduit, and metaphor, for such an expose'. The price shines through the most direct orifice, as Dave constantly reassures them that the tapes are only for "me, myself and I" and makes plans to see the whore again for another shot, as soon as possible, and just after they've had a really big meal. "When do you usually go?"

From volume #3:

The first girl: Lisa is short, very fat and like most of the whores throughout the series, hispanic. She has a huge belly that is slashed across into lolling plump bulges by a thick crease that could be a deep scar, too tight pants line or just horribly unnatural.

The second girl: In the room at the same time as Lisa, another hispanic. Wears dark blue satin panties and a cheap shiny black top. She answers to the name: Baby. Slick wet jeri-curl formed and molded and fused two tone (orange-blonde to her neck and down her back, pitch black on top) hair.

She tries to shit into a popcorn bowl and presses hard into her fat puffed distended asshole. She's skinny and boney and dark skinned. Says she hasn't gone in two weeks.

Dave tells both girls to stand next to each other, turn around, bend over and spread. Baby says "just like when we were in jail".

The third girl: Amy, whom David calls a "strawberry blonde" and explains outloud "has a beautiful daughter and she's gonna see her tomorrow but right now she needs a little money".

Amy has slurred speech and repeatedly asks Dave not to film her face or the tattoo just above her cunt of her boyfriend's full name. "This is just for me, not for anyone else" and then Dave asks if that's the name of her pimp.

You've been pregnant before, besides your first child?

"Yeah, I had a miscarriage."

Well, that's a drag ...how long ago was that?

"About three months ago ...almost like the time I lost my daughter."

And:

"I usually have a tan line, but I haven't been wearing shorts because I got all these, you know, bruises."

The fourth girl: Wedda; thin worn muscle and tendoned look to her thirty-one year old body.

"I try to stay healthy."

And:

"Alot of girls are just 24–7 out there on the

street, I try to give time for myself."

The fifth girl: Patty. Blonde Mexican trash looks beat up Irish. Eating pizza and drinking coronas on Dave's balcony with her friend Diane, another hispanic pig in wide mirrored shades and frizzed out afro-mop like a fright wig.

Dave talks about his bad luck getting the whores to give him the big thick logs of shit he wants.

"Well, sometimes drugs constipates you", Patty slurs then explains that she takes drugs in the morning and it definitely effects her bowel movements, it "makes 'em big, makes my butt bleed."

And:

"I wake up kinda sick cause I need to, you know, do my drugs."

And:

"I was with a girl for six years. That was my wife. She's like a boy. But actually she's a woman. She thinks she's a man."

Patty wants the money before she tries to shit.

"Half and half. What we agreed on, first."

Her ass is wide and flabby and dotted with picked sores and zits. Scratches and indentations and cuts and red marks cover her entire whore's section of ass, thighs and lumpy waist.

The sixth girl: Diane the fright wig, also has a go at shitting but is as unsuccessful as all the others. Her ass is elephant flabby and hung loose low unto her legs like great mounds of old wet rolled up and chewed garbage carpet. Cellulite cheesed and pock marked with absolutely no muscle or snap except within a thick protruding varicose vein or two. Just hung and sick and whored wobbly meat flabs of dead flesh.

In Volume #5, Joanne leaves Dave in the bedroom to go smoke crack in the kitchen.

"I always have a rock when I get home."

Patty returns in this volume, shares a smoke with Joanne and continues to cough up phlegm:

"Yeah, that's what that shit does to your lungs."

In Volume #11, dedicated entirely to two girls: Kristy and Toni, both rather young looking and acting – possibly less than the eighteen years required by law. Kristy, in particular acts childish; bouncing around and posing her fat belly, huge ass and little firm tits, talking about her mother and, after a brief stab at licking Toni's wide open cunt, asking her how she did.

She may also be retarded.

David asks Toni: How long have you had a bush like that? When did you start growing hair down there?

"About 4 or 5 years ago," she mutters and poses with her hands behind her black hair.

Toni wants to see the video.

Kristy digs at the shit in her asshole by reaching two fingers deeply into her cunt.

Dave gets especially smarmy in this edition, due most probably to the girls' youth. He couldn't get away with repeatedly kissing all the other older hookers the way he does Toni. He also probably wouldn't want to.

"Rodney Moore, the extraordinary 'King Of Cream', returns with another soaking wet edition of Creme De La Face, the video series for anyone who loves to see pretty girl's faces continuously splattered with huge helpings of jism."

(CREME DE LA FACE #5; JUST FOR THE CUM OF IT, 2 hours, Odyssey Group Video.)

"Take a look at this one boys. This is a west coast shot series of local hookers shitting all over. This series starts with #3 because 1 & 2 are pretty ruff, but they get better each tape. In fact, as I type this description up I have been informed #4 is complete and being forwarded to me. This series was started by some brown lovers like yourself who would like to produce good quality viewable movies instead of multi generation tapes that are almost impossible to tell which end it is coming out of. This is intended to be a constantly evolving project with a movie expected every 2-3 weeks. We have subscribed to this project and will carry the entire series. As far as I know we are the only commercial source selling them. Call shooter if you would like to subscribe to this series and receive them as they are released. Go ahead order this one. See if it's what you like. Remember they only get better."
(BROWN BOMBER, advertised in private catalog)

"In December 1985 Martin received a call from Lou Ellen Couch's sister. LuLu had been stabbed to death in a street fight while defending a friend. Her last words were 'Tell Martin and Mary Ellen LuLu died'."
(STREETWISE; PHOTOGRAPHS BY MARY ELLEN MARK, Mary Ellen Mark, Aperture, 1985)

"Just before a police sergeant announced that Alice was stabbed to death by a 28 year old Latin male, and Alice's prostitute roomie explained that her murderer used an 8" long 2" wide butcher knife, Alice herself was interviewed about her future:

"'I predict that I'll still be with Harold, um, probably, well, I don't know, if age catches up with me fast, I might not be doing this but, you know, as of now, yeah, I'll probably still, you know, walk the streets.'"
(HOOKER, Directed by Robert Niemark, 79 minutes, 1985)

See also Jennie Livingston's PARIS IS BURNING, John-Paul Davidson's THE BOYS FROM BRAZIL, Nick Broomfield's HEIDI FLIESS: HOLLYWOOD MADAM and AILEEN WOURNOS: THE SELLING OF A SERIAL KILLER, Kate Davis' GIRLTALK, Playboy's DOROTHY STRATTEN, THE UNTOLD STORY, Frontline's DEATH OF A PORN STAR, America Undercover's HIGH ON CRACK STREET, Bill Kurtis' NEW YORK STREET SEX and DYING FOR SEX, CNN's FACES OF SLAVERY, and, especially:

"I bought a rice farm for Aoi and I left Thailand. One year later I went back but she was not there. I found her working in Bangkok, in a sleazy massage parlour called 'The Happy House'. I asked her why and she said 'It is my fate'."
(GOOD WOMAN OF BANGKOK, directed by Dennis O'Rourke, 90 minutes, 1993)

"This video captures women going to the bathroom in the privacy of the ladies room. Great patience and risk went into its making, and the connoisseur of ladies room voyeurism will surely enjoy it.

"This presentation captures another

thirty or so women with their panties down. CLR-3 was filmed in both B & W and in color. A past review precedes and an interesting Candid Ladies Room EDITFEST follows. Enjoy!"
(CANDID LADIES ROOM, CLR-3, 90 minutes)

"The trash bin had been emptied Monday morning, police said, and there was no garbage in it when the fully clothed body was discovered."
(WOMAN FOUND DEAD IN TRASH BEHIND SCHOOL, Chicago Tribune, April 25, 1996)

It doesn't have to be this way. You don't have to be this ugly. The troll everyone knows – short and fat dyed dirty hair all colors of penny boxed blonde and black and hard grey, old Irish pig squashed white wisconsin stupidity – doesn't have to exist this way.
  You don't have to drink. You don't have to be addicted like trash. You don't have to lie to your drug friends and co-workers, your johns and your pimp that way. You don't have to be so fucking defensive.
  Who fucked you up this way?
  Let's get rid of the excuses and armor and that ratty thick shell of hate that makes your natural attributes – beauty – so fucking anally perverse. How can your sore toothless face with all those pocks and blemishes and bruises ever retain any of the parent imbued bad luck you were raised with? Do you think that by slithering underneath all that make-up and attitude and stumbling slow chemical drowse that you can hide the great series of mistakes that has sent you right down here

now?

    Do you know the market for you, right now? Do you know you were fucking born for this? Asking for it? Just waiting ...waiting and begging for it?

    Come on; who fucked you up this way?

    Don't you dare say a name. Don't even think to find a whoever and struggle around tweezing it out of that wrinkled fried matterless mess. Don't make another sound unless that belch points directly back at you and all your petty problems. I don't think EKG machines can register the brain waves of cows these days. They're man-made beasts now. Totally inorganic lumps that could probably grow square in cardboard boxes if it made sense economically, and wouldn't frighten the public aesthetically. What sort of farmyard raised you, dear? What small sort of mistakes were made back at the farmhouse? Now, slowly, gather what brain cells you have left to pop and press from the diaphragm up: Who fucked you up this bad? What kind of sick lifeless pig turned you into this mess?

    You know it wasn't anybody else, don't you? Don't you and your young-ish sore cunt truly know that: when you blur on the plain mat ceiling above all those jabbing discharging cocks, needles and jagged fingers? What part of the new age was lost on you? What part of some equitable inclusive self negating pop philosophy did you miss? What created that hole your entire existence fell into? What classes did you skip? What kind of help did you forget to get?

    What kind of person – fuck, I know you was simple country folk – could you be without all the excuses you sell so well you don't remember you even started. Inside that burning chipping greying brain where you barker out a brand new cut of pig; just behind that drunk lost slosh and slipped veneer of protection and raw advertising insecurity, peeled open asshole bloody, lies the answer the prosecutor needs to find.

How can you change? What will you offer later as to what good you can do now? What can you afford to sell or buy or what is it you prefer at this particular stem of uncluttered hallucination? Inside that splintered and re-plastered rotten barrel lies a thick hardened fistule of lard and fecal disease cancer and bodily quim cum and blood formed flesh that has your DNA red stamped all over it.

That beast – this special little idea – never fucking existed. And the jury fucking know it. And the prosecutor, who already got paid, spat the garish cheap advertising through her teeth so easily it bothered even her; for a second or two:

No one, I'm sure, has to tell you this. None of this – these details, these motives, these actions and defense excuses – has to be explained to you. Or anybody. As wrong. As intrinsically evil or, if you prefer, as absolutely anti everything humans are destined to do, want or accomplish. That these acts which naturally repel; naturally – that is, viscerally, immediately disgust down to the very roots of one's soul – these acts are unbearable. These acts against someone else, whether you believe in god or a higher power or buddha or just your parents or love in a hard, hard unforgiving world, are decidedly evil. They are incorrect. They are loathsome. They are destructive. They are needless. They are selfish and worthless and sickeningly hurtful. Self-obsessed, vacant acts that are an affront to everyone – everyone that understands themselves as part of a community or a family or a thinking individual as part of a chain that includes everyone working together, helping, struggling, commiserating, sharing and protecting each other for as long as we're here on earth.

These acts hurt more than just the victim, who in certain hateful base eyes is seen just as a plaything; a toy without feelings or emotions or reasons or plans or place. These shameful acts mortally harm us all. Because it takes away a great deal of our humanity. Some of what we call life. These acts cast a pall over our lives and transform us into less than we were. They deplete our resources, gnaw away at our hope and trust and concern and compassion and rip and stomp and steal our faith and future.

These acts offer nothing. They consume our time and energy. They pillage and waste, they raze and burn and leave nothing whatsoever in the smoke and blood and pain. Not even for the selfish damaged individual so sick in himself, so low and degraded and torpid and mad.

These acts make no sense. Not even to him. Any acknowledgement of basic, rudimentary workings of compassion or empathy or humanity, if there is even the most remote possibility that those concepts can be located anywhere here at all, is only evident in the calculated twisting and circumvention of such feelings in the victim. All victims are innocent. None deserve their pain. No one deserves to be hurt. No one asks for terror and force and control and bruises and blood and frightened last screaming seconds and years of tortured flesh and mind destroyed insanity.

No. Feelings don't exist here. They couldn't.

Not here, not as bludgeons; not this way. These definitions are all inadequate.

So we are left with a new reality predicated on immediate blind lust and personal drives bent and sick on destruction and cruelty. And anything we knew previous – anything else that was important to us, that was special or meaningful or purposeful like family and concern for our fellow man and charity and realized dreams – is now complete garbage. Rendered to filth. Vain vacuous chimeras.

No, we can't let that happen. We can't look for understanding here. As humans, as people who seek to produce and help instead of destroy and steal and rape, we try to look for the boy that was instead of the man who is. We try desperately to cling to some semblance of ourselves, some greater knowledge of our position here in nature and see what went wrong; what exactly could have turned something so inexplicably terribly wrong against us. What did he do. What did we do. How can we help.

We are naturally inclined to look down at the lifeless scorched earth left in his wake and pick for clues. Because we feel incomplete. Our need to understand and feel a sense of unity, of oneness, of brotherhood, of love, of the universal mother; all changed now. All reduced invalid. All of us left with nothing rooted, just a big black of empty. Of dust. And a sad miserable reality that nothing can ever be the same again. Everything shot right to fucking hell.

All of us: robbed. Soulless. Dead. All of us murdered.

No one wants to say these words. One is forced to.

We are the family that suffers the loss of a very special part of ourselves – an unreplaceable gem of promise and hope; the victim from which all this cannibalistic hatred and harm and pain spirals ever outward. We are now condemned to the reality of this animal's design, his whim and reaction and illness. We are now formed in his image.

The shattered humanity of everyone but his.

When you see that video. And you see that beautiful girl with the beautiful blonde hair and bright clear eyes and freshly buffed up rosey cheeks; look to see what she becomes. And see if we don't become the same. See if it doesn't kill all of us. Because she changes right there on that tape. Gradually over the span of twenty filmed minutes that the camera focuses on her. Watch her become less than nothing, watch her body drain and empty and die and see the it she becomes as her new god, the creator of us all, fills up inside her vulnerable little body.

This then is the new age. This is the second fucking coming. This animal that fed her cocaine and filthy lies and easy answers from easier money; this is what creeps into her marketable body before he allows her blood to oil over the carpeted floor and silk bedsheets in their bedroom, before he uses her up and lets her rot away from him. Used and dirtied and now worn and no longer worth even one extra phonecall minute.

That penis she places in her mouth. And all the cocks she sucks. Isn't his. The man in this particular twenty minutes that pumps and grinds and pushes his erection into her vagina and paws at her breasts and finally ejaculates onto her back; having divested himself of friction in every human hole she owned and sold, is not the god that killed her. That big hard-on cock was a hired stupid pawn stud – a substitute cock in the greater fuck. Told what to do. Paid for his time, his pleasure, his complicity in her all too available death.

    She hugs him afterwards. Cum still soaking into her milk-fed soft skin and sliding down her spine and puddling onto her round, over eighteen, butt. She kisses him and he pulls her tighter. A job well done.

    A job now over and filmed forever for the god to use, to keep, to store and sell and show his friends and impress or talk about and prove or just masturbate to.

    You can pause the video now. He can stop the film on exactly the frame he likes best. That gentle devil tongue on the red tip of a fat whore cock, his hairy scrotum pushed up rough against her midwestern peach complexion and heroin zits.

    On her face.

    Cock inside her mouth. Up her vagina, as her thin meaty cunt lips pull apart and hang slippery low around that bull thick fat veined hard-on that shoves up deeper and deeper as she squats down lower and lower onto all of that paid sweaty mindless animal action.

    On her objectified skinny well formed body.

    Nice tits, firm teen type rump.

    Blonde bush untrimmed but clean.

    Soft lips and endearing smile that stays throughout the entire mouth fucking dog licking blow-job.

    It's all right there.

    And it's all there in the right place now. The robotic instructions and angles, the tedious gropes and thrusts and facial expressions. All of it is brand new in the new heaven; the new aeon of the young selfish god. It's all real now. Reality has become fiction before this. This twenty minute of dumb teen approximations, fantasy fucking and cunt lapping and cocksucking and dick cumming and hair held back so we could see her natural tits heft and fall with every rutting good long powerhouse slam is now the holy fucking bible.

No one need be ashamed now.

You don't even need a safe word now.

No one needs a second thought.

You can see real sex roll right before you. That cock in her mouth must be remarkably similar to the gun she placed there just a few days later.

How proud her boss must be.

Her god practically predicted it. Fucking walked on water to show us all he knew about everything.

Imagine that gun sliding and pumping out of her steadied mouthed head as that gorilla with the smaller dirtier smellier flesh fucks her face. Freeze on that skin and muscle throbbing vein, hard and tight and firm against her padded pink tongue, and that quick last taste of black finished smooth hot steel and fingered wood and a trigger that drug limp pulled back quicker than a brain pulse.

That cum close-up trickles like a small amount of blood. But not as well. Not as full-bodied and viscus and perfect pump seep spill and spread and soak beneath the plush colored clothes into the floorboards. You can really jack off to the crime scene photos now. All that head and face and bullethole splashed behind and to the side of the large bed.

If she coughed on pre-cum. Just a little. Just a little piss or a little sick discharge. Fuck. The way her skinny lungs filled with the warm red blood from her collapsing throat and shoulders. Fuck the way he grew hard in her head and jerked his ass muscles to feel the inside of her warm sloppy face that ripped and tore and fell apart and peeled and splattered and came and prayed.

    Nothing better than a paid fuck on cocaine cunt. Nothing better than a new cunt to fuck every night, in your own home, alone at night, holding your cock in front of the TV scattered images moving each way inside a single little hand held orgasm.

    Messy and yet as clean as can be.

    Tonight it's her face split into two.

    Yesterday it was her little jiggling tits and hard pink nipples pert and unbruised. Covered in caked blood and that little twitch of slightly pained belly I didn't catch before.

    Tomorrow it'll be the humiliation of the money shot brought home to mom. Back in the cheap seats, mom; does dad still want to fuck the hole that produced the thing he saw fuck anything with enough cash, drugs or connections. The god himself said fuck this one just for the camera and she was more than happy.

    And what part of the little porno body reminded you of the one you owned not so long ago and grew ape hard even just thinking about it.

    Dad can't pretend now. Can't deny. Neither can mom or the cops or the nigger welfare jury and job hunting prosecution.

    God has made everything real.

    Everything is clear.

    And no one wants to hear it. No one wants any of it. No one wants to see the photos and the film that effortlessly combines post-mortem and pre-mortem into a whole new exciting religion. No one wants the proof. No one wants to be here for this; any of it.

No one wants this to happen. No one wants the possibility of this to exist – not to themselves or those – anyone – around them.

And no one deserves this. No matter what. No one deserves to be anywhere near these actions or the descriptions – the pornographic details – of these acts. Words, thoughts, dreams made flesh, evidence. No one asked for any of this filth.

No one needs their reactions explained. You don't have to investigate what you already know to be naturally, instinctively beneath you. You already know exactly what happened. And what's wrong with all of it.

And nothing has changed. No matter how much this motherfucker has tried.

These things don't change.

And I'm sorry to have had to add to this sort of noise, this sort of filth, this sort of demeaning consideration. And to have had to drag you all along, when you already knew, and didn't ask to be here and would rather be anywhere else. I'm sorry, just truly sorry, for all of it.

1. CREME DE LA FACE #12; PRETTY FACES TO CUM ON, 2 hours, Odyssey Group Video.

THREE

"Without me, those crimes could probably not have been committed. It was I who was instrumental in procuring the children, children who would more readily accompany strangers if they were a woman and a man than they would a man on his own."
(MYRA HINDLEY: MY STORY, Myra Hindley, *The Guardian*, December 18, 1995)

"I slept terribly last night. I should be used to it now. That dream has haunted me day and night for 25 years."
(FOR THE LOVE OF LESLEY, Ann West, W.H. Allen, 1989)

Wizard, the shit eater from *You Said A Mouthful* (Slave & Master) returned in *The Bizarre Debut Of Mistress Anne* (also Slave & Master), this time, to chew on and suck out a heavy flowed blood soaked tampon pulled slowly from a goth whore's fat meat folded deep red cunt.
      Slave & Master videos used to be available through Bijou Video in Chicago until an agreement was reached between the Bijou's owner and vice police not to sell them anymore.
      Mistress Anne, not as interesting as Wizard

unfortunately, continued to make bondage and torture videos – a great many of them sadly cartoonish; though that's what the market and law called for. Mole Video in downstate Illinois attempted to carry as much as they could of old (even then) fat wrinkled dyed blonde Mistress Anne's oeuvre until they too ceased to be, due to police pressure.

Superlive of Ronkonkoma, NY, used to publish a "Catalogue Of Brown And Gold Erotica", among their specialty stock, that featured the scowling Mistress Anne sat atop a naked slave's face on the front cover.

Mistress Anne, it seems, started to make her reputation in scat films during the very early eighties: rather along the lines of her forcing her willing, paying, fat middle-aged closet bottom to eat her shit.

A store in Chicago will sell some of these old tapes in badly dubbed form, in Memorex boxes even, for $100.00 a crack. Cut up descriptions from old catalogs are taped to other blank video boxes and displayed along the walls. An old prick with cataracts, who works behind the counter shoeless – no doubt due to his old war corns – is quick to explain how he hasn't seen any of these films and has no interest in seeing them either.

You can select from six or so films playing constantly in the peep booths along the side wall for a quarter for about a minute and a half.

If you're looking for shit. And shit eaters and shitters and shit fuckers and pissers and piss swallowers, you have very few choices. You simply have to take expensive chances.

The current reissues of old Christopher Rage films have been re-edited and contain little of their original appeal. Even the more adventuresome gay-identified/alternative porn purveyors are unwilling to involve themselves in the scat market, seeing as arrests for obscenity are so costly to fight and easy to bring.

SVE has a series that collects the loops of the Seventies onto compilation videos titled *Grinders*. Each edition lasts around sixty minutes and contains badly reproduced photos from just a few of the included loops on the xeroxed covers. No names or titles or other descriptions, apparently, necessary.

Just search the racks for the small grainy stills of hanging mamas' bellies splashed with cum. Or a long haired whore squeezing her nipples clamp tight to release a messy sprinkler system of filthy lactose.

Diamond's Period from Diamond Productions has the title star, thin and young and availably made up, dragging around inside her swollen puffed and red stained cunt with a vibrator. Her well hung close cropped young co-star laps at her cunt in a later scene, before sliding his cock into the stinking sticking mess. He pulls out of her to jerk his only barely red tinted cock off on her ass and boney back. She goes down on him and his questionable hygiene. And none of it is as messy or gory or, even, clear as obsessive fans of all that is performed and required by the monstrously clumsy ballet called Creation and womb worn entropy would hope. Or imagine.

Diamond's drawn cheeks pop and her ass bags flop and her ribs and thighbones jut through her skinny fatless flesh. Like all mothers, potential or declining, she wears far too much make-up to be fully resplendent in all things natural. Rather like a suburban make-out teen turned obvious.

Blood dots and smears her friend's cock, but looks only like the faint lipstick blow-job aftermath left by most nigger or mexican porno stars. Blood speckles around her thin trimmed cunt and pubic hair but never blots the sheets in puddles or close up drips. The way your wife would probably do if she didn't jam a diaper up herself before she laid down to bed every thirty or so days. The vibrator manned by Diamond to slut around inside of her creeping dying walls is used to display the deep clot color of her blood and its viscousness.

The men who come into the Chicago shop with the shit videos are mostly older gentlemen. Many of these men will squeeze their way into your peep booth on just the slightest offer of attention or acquiescence.

These old men continue to suck cock. And they seem to like to make you cum. Some jerk themselves off, many don't even bother. They suck at your cock like a machine, like a teat, like a dottering old wheezing man whose wife died of a brain aneurysm long ago and this is as close as they get to flesh these days. Like they were sucking their own.

They haven't always been queer.

They've been in public showers before without getting hard or even thinking about it.

Whores are too drugged and money hungry these days. Cars are unavailable on their pension plan. These stores are heterosexually oriented somehow.

And one quickly generates a perverse – seemingly perverse; easily and lazily labeled perverse – interest in seeing these old bags' sunken drooped lifeless cocks. Their dying bodies.

There are chairs half way down the steps at The Bijou just in case some of the older clientele need a breather on the way up or down.

These old men will lick out your asshole if you turn around.

Their cocks will get semi-hard, or surprise you by getting very hard and quite often enough they themselves or you can make them ejaculate.

Somewhere, that's what they want. To cum. An orgasm. A release. Some pleasure.

But none of them wanted any of this. Not this way. No matter what they have to do. Or what they get into their now rotten minds about what they miss or the shit they want to watch, the period they want to smell, the damage they want to track. The mothering they want to feast on and own and sell and beat into fleshless dust.

None of them really want what they get.

Since my arrest for possession of child pornography back in 1985 I have been very careful. The last batch of kiddie porn I bought was in Japan last year but I was sure to leave my purchases in the hands of a friend when I left. As it was, I spent three hours in customs with up to four different agents all poring over whatever items I figured I could bring through legally. *Death Women* caused alot of concern but eventually passed.

My favorite photos from this last batch were of peep shots taken of little children who were unaware of, or unconcerned with, the photographer. A little girl, no more than maybe seven years old, helping her mother paint a wall, her loose dago t-shirt hanging wide open at her skinny armpit exposing a tiny brown nipple. Lots of shots of schoolgirls in traditional – Western catholic type – school uniforms playing and running and tumbling so that their dresses hitch up over their clean tight mommy picked fresh white panties. And swimming shots of tight pre-teen vagina curves and slick butt cracks and protruding hard girl flat tit nipples barely underneath sopping wet skin slim bathing trunk material. And surreptitious bathroom peeks: just a bit more than little babies really but older soft firm butts squatting down, away from their mothers and friends for seconds only, over those horrible Japanese concrete toilets in the floor.

More graphic depictions of sex acts between all combinations and ages were cleanly available and waded through. But what I liked of the new explosion in peep videos and magazines was the clear intentions of the photographer. The flesh – supposedly innocent, or at least ignorant – becomes conduit. It is only what is directed on to it.

The best photos of the sixteen children massacred in Dunblane, Scotland by Thomas Hamilton were collected and published in *Paris Match* (28 Mars 1996). All the news shows here in the States carried footage of the ever widening floral bed created in front of the school as well as weeping, howling, hand hiding mothers and, of course, film segments from Hamilton's large collection showing him teaching and manhandling his young shirtless charges over a gymhorse.

In color shots with the children's faces digitized out, *Paris Match* froze one of the video stills for a perfect view of the boney body clad, only, in baggy shorts and gym-shoes and socks that Hamilton loved so much. Another snap of him posing with the boys from one of his many scout troops shows his smile, confidence amid the right age – all clothed in t-shirts and jerseys except one boy sitting in the front, shirtless, blond, and the smallest one there.

LE MONSTRE
    Déjà en 1989, des mères pourchassaient le pervers dans la rue.[1]
    I can't read French. The cover of the issue is all sixteen then live, now dead children, including the eleven girls he didn't fucking care for, in nice cropped close ups on glossy stock.
    KEVIN, 5 ANS
    DAVID, 5 ANS
    BRETT, 6 ANS
    JOHN, 5 ANS
    ROSS, 5 ANS
    The information came first.

"There was talk of boys having to parade around in boxer shorts and puff out their chests for inspection, of hundreds of photographs, taken and of bullying and fondling at his camps."
(WHY?, *The Sunday Times*, 17 March 1996)

"He then took a bus back to his special flat, perhaps to spend the evening watching one of the hundreds of the videos he had made of 'his boys', most aged between eight and twelve, filmed semi-naked, flexing their muscles."
(THE LAST DAYS OF THOMAS HAMILTON, *Sunday Telegraph*, 17 March 1996)

"Many parents complained to authorities about his penchant for photographing the boys bare-chested and for fondling and bullying the youths in his charge."

(INNOCENTS LOST, *People*, April 1, 1996)

"There were 20 to 30 young boys wearing only swimming trunks, parading as if they were in a fashion show."
(THE SORDID MISFIT OBSESSED BY GUNS, *International Express*, 20 March–26 March, 1996)

"The pictures of bare chested boys on his walls could be seen by anyone looking in his window; a woman neighbor was shown his collection of videos of boys running around his Loch Lomond camp as if they were the most natural thing in the world for a youth leader to film."
(THE LIFE AND DEATH OF THOMAS WATT HAMILTON, *The Independent On Sunday*, 17 March 1996)

"They told me he was taking lots of photographs throughout and later they all went to sleep in the same bed."
(THEY HAD SO MANY CHANCES TO STOP THE MONSTER, *News Of The World*, 17 March 1996)

"Tom always blamed the parents for failing to provide their children with wholesome diets. He was always talking about healthy bodies leading to healthy minds."
(I COULD KILL FOUR PEOPLE WITH A SINGLE BULLET, *The Mail On Sunday*, 17 March 1996)

The girls' names could be used to place little fake personalities to the pictures one might masturbate with, to, in the comfort of one's bathroom, say, in

Tokyo, just five minutes away from the most lovely family owned and immaculate Kiddie Porn stockist.

Particularly recommended, and up market even, is the easily available *Alice Club* which runs down and captures all the happenings in kidnews, in Japanese and full color and perfectly clear black and white, monthly.

Say you don't like Japanese flesh. You're just this much more interested in something a bit closer to home.

        CHARLOTTE, 5 ANS
        EMILY, 5 ANS
        ABIGAIL, 5 ANS
        JOANNA, 5 ANS
        EMMA, 5 ANS
        SOPHIE, 5 ANS
        MHAIRI, 5 ANS
        HANNAH, 5 ANS
        MEGAN, 5 ANS
        MELISSA, 5 ANS
        VICTORIA, 5 ANS

Video shops catering to a large gay clientele have recently been getting away with Dutch and German transfers of barely legal porn. In Chicago, at least. Boys just over or at legal age who look young are the excuses; the chance that the boys are younger and lying is the market. Though all have pubic hair and big, thick and too grown (no matter what the ethnicity) cocks.

        ACTION BOY
        BOYS FOR SALE
        GERO GAY EXTRA
        SEXY MOTEL
        SMILING BOYS
        MEGA BOYS: MESSAGE BOYS
        TEENANGEL #5

**IMAGE EURO PRESENTS: DAS SPRITZ HOTEL
SPERMA MEN #36
EIN VERFICKTER UMZUG**

It seems that around that age – eighteen or so – boys can get away with more than girls. The market is bigger for that sort of youth look, in boys (the term "boys" alone has a much wider application than does its female counterpart), as well as being harder to judge age in thin, drawn and wasted rough trade misfit hustler types.

But there's no reason to work all that hard. To deliberately fool yourself. That specific interest is easy to come by.

"Three months of hopeful waiting ended in anguish for Jimmy Ryce's family Saturday, when police found the missing 9 year old's mutilated remains and charged a Dade handyman with the killing."
(MISSING BOY SLAIN, DISMEMBERED, *The Tampa Tribune- Times*, December 10, 1995)

"Nobody knows. Nobody can ever know the hell this family has been through, and will go through forever."
(WHAT IS LEFT TO FEEL AFTER RYCE TRAGEDY, Gary Stein, commentary, *Sun-Sentinel*, December 10, 1995)

"The end was more horrific than anything they had imagined. But, at least, Don and Claudine Ryce know what happened to their little boy."
(I KNOW HE'S IN HEAVEN, *Sun-Sentinel*, December 10, 1995)

"Moulton said her ex-husband was driving around the area, hoping to find his son. She said he was 'very distraught and upset'".
(PAROLED KILLER QUESTIONED ON MISSING BOY, *Chicago Sun-Times*, August 11, 1995)

"'Chris, we are never going to stop looking for you until we find you', Moulton said, breaking down into tears. 'If I can take any of the pain for you, I will do that. I am doing my best to take your pain so you don't have to suffer.'"
(MOM: WE ARE NEVER GOING TO STOP LOOKING, *Chicago Sun-Times*, August 13, 1995)

"His grave was a plywood board and a dusting of dirt so thin a foot was sticking out, an awful, unfair end for a child who set out only to fish on a lazy summer afternoon."
(SEARCH ENDS WITH A GRIM DISCOVERY, *Chicago Sun-Times*, August 16, 1995)

"The photo is now etched in our minds: eager, trusting blue eyes: a broad, gap-toothed smile; neatly combed blonde hair, dimples pushed in by his grin."
(BEHIND THE SMILE: A BOY WHO WAS LOVED BY ALL, *Chicago Sun-Times*, August 18, 1995)

"He waited there for quite awhile until the small blue casket was covered with dirt. He waited, friends said, 'to make sure Christopher was in his grave and safe.'"
(SLAIN BOY IS MOURNED AS PICTURE OF INNOCENCE, *Chicago Sun-Times*, August 23, 1995)

Sex has everything to do with age. Even more than infection. With waste and depletion and entropy. Everything after. There is no such thing as a clean fuck.

Sex is a matter of degrees. It's a history of options. When sex is pornography, it is born of safety and privilege.

The formula is slow and reactionary. It is functional and ugly. The deviations that seem more investigative; more dangerous and difficult and spiritual and thus, more honest than mere urge or instinct are, in fact, the very same thing. Manifest confusion. Dedicated self-aggrandizement. They are not perversions. They are not truthful. They are not naked. They are not education. You fuck yourself no matter what you're looking for, find or settle on. No matter what you say. No matter what you believe.

I'm bad at guessing ages. I have a very dear video of these little girls. *Gymnastics: Coaching And Spotting Gymnasts* put out by a little company in Florida for, I guess, budding coaches and the mothers of the little featurettes. There are seven little girls. All in those little danskin outfits that stick right up in, on and across all the places you knew it should. The coach, some blond muscle head wad, talks the camera through the correct way to hold the girls as they bend, flip, stretch, jog and wiggle on a wooden beam and then some padded blue mats. He palms their backs and waists and supports their tight little asses and barely brushes their flat boney chests. I imagine they're between six and nine, though they could be just slightly younger. I hope they're not older but it would be possible. Their smiles are genuine. Their smirks and studied concentration pose; all the same. Their hair looks decidedly mommy primped. Their sex is all in their perfect trim asses and straight chests and that firm space between their spread legs as just a line of shadow or strained bent-over thought. This particular video is very matter of fact and only fifteen minutes long. What I know of little girls who're older is what leads me to my guess at their ages.

I know there's this little girl, age eleven only, who used to sleep in the nude. Used to sleep upstairs in her parents' house, in her large perfectly kept bed in her immaculate bedroom, alone, nude and dark.

At eleven she was wearing make-up. Her body was just starting to develop. Into whatever will happen over the next five or six or ten uncomfortable years.

The girls in the video don't wear make-up. They have white hand powder splashed about little corners of their bodies, some on their tiny sport butts, others across their chests and crotches. But their lips and eyebrows, their eyes and baby cheeks are all their own color. All their own. One little girl on the cover of the video (showing all seven girls in a clumsy smiling pyramid, posing, supporting and leaning child careful), down on her hands and knees on the right corner, looks to be developing a little quicker. But this may be due to the way she slumps her back rather than anything else more natural. Budding hurtful motherhood. Just not yet.

Many gymnasts train so hard that their bodies stall puberty. Menarche can, in extreme cases, begin in their twenties at the cessation of their rigorous training schedules. The girls' bodies are left and kept in a frozen pre-pubescent state: brittle bones and low estrogen and skinny womanless muscle.

The eleven year old had to crawl downstairs to her parents' bedroom and scream at them: tell them she was raped and show them the blood. Tell them about the window and how dark it was and how he, first, tickled her feet with a knife.

How could it have felt. Are you alright now sweetheart? Do you need a while alone? Do you need to cry it all out – it's alright, now, it's alright, would you like to be held? Darling. My poor baby.

Did the fuck she had pinch tight every muscle in her body like stretched fucking wood? Like muscle hard flesh gymnasts develop and desire? Or did you just feel the pain inside your body like any little girl losing her virginity would. Inside all over; not easy to forget, burning to piss everything out.

I watched my sister grow up. I have a video of her talking to my mother – my mom behind the camera. My sister looks like she's talking directly to me.

Just her head and shoulders, clad in a fuzzy black sweater. She has a cute pageboy cut of black hair that forms a neat flat helmet around her just pre-teen chubby face. A gentle small nose stubs out below somewhat sunken though flawless dark eyes. Thin lips all pinched inside a clean peach complexion flattened out by a bad video dub. She doesn't smile. She's mad about something. There's no sound. And it is just of her face, I think, from around twelve years old.

I remember watching her masturbating.

She was squatting in a bathtub only a quarter filled with tepid grey water. She was patting her vagina, perched up on her haunches, one hand steadying her gangly deformed weight on the side porcelain of the tub, the other rubbing between her legs. Like a monkey, a fatty ape, a stupid dead to the world selfish hog.

I'm watching from the back. I can't see her face or her cunt. I move a little to see her bent forward boney back and the sides of her thin pubescent stomach rolls. I focus on the crack of her ass that peeks up as her shoulder moves to tell me she's feeling herself.

She just had her period, perhaps.

Or she's decided it feels good to do that. To pet and caress her hairing cunt. But she doesn't know better than to just slap at it.

Would you like someone else to do that? Do you even realize the possibility? Do you understand sharing, or getting that close. Do you understand the difference between rape and just a fuck that you yourself want, asked for, wondered about, lusted after. Caught. Mounted. Deposited. Wiped off. Do you know what your body can do to your brain, can you comprehend anything like this?

I mean; would you mind?

Did your face flush, your belly tighten, nipples harden and did you cum? And how will that change?

When you're thirteen. When you were just a teenager. When you're of legal age. When you hit forty. When you're finally given over to your oldest child's home to exist, in the way and hated, over a birthday cake then and again or a nice dress dropped off at the Goodwill.

You liked it when mommy washed your hair. When you were just so little and inoffensive.

And now you know you like that special place that you found when you're bathing.

You can tell me.

I saw you.

You don't know what you're playing with. You didn't know what you started.

I've seen bodies like yours. I know what you'll be. I saw what was aching to happen even then. Tits like yours sag like the ones on the pig I fucked when I was looking for pigs to fuck. The fleshy spread, the slithery grasps and cowering slides. Your shrill embarrassment. Your stumbling mistakes again and again. I watched you grow and turn and form and fail. I remember that age very well. It took a long time.

Nine year old Amber was in Girl Scouts, of course, and during the first week of cookie sales, she was pulled from the little bike she was riding and stuffed into an old black pick-up.

She lived in Arlington, Texas, had blue eyes and was wearing pink jeans and a grey shirt with multicolored handprints splashed all over it on the last day of her life. She wore her lovely brown hair in a cute little nine year old ponytail.

Amber's mother, the day of Amber's abduction, cried:

"I want to get out there and do something. I want to get out there on the street and holler and holler for her. I know that's not going to do anything, but I just want her back.

Just drop her off. Let her walk home by herself. Just don't hurt my baby."[2]

The video has changed though there is really nothing new. Nothing different. It remains as exactly as I see it. It is nothing more than that.

Amber was found dead in a ditch.

Sisters bleed into mothers if you let them.

It all starts to look the same then. It is the

same.

A mid-twenties/middle-aged thing sold me a video of her daughter. The video, police and child rights advocates will be pleased to know, was only of a three or four year old girl playing at some beach. Some grey but sunny, sandy though rough, cheap and hot beach near, I think, filthy but playable Lake Michigan. The baby wore a chintzy lovely little bathing suit – one piece wrapped snug to too tight around her tiny bunched up chub ill-formed child's body. At all times. The video lasts a bit over a half an hour and it, honestly, is just as innocent as you can imagine.

I thought it might be a good idea if the thing filmed herself changing the girly's diapers or helping it into that stretched out sling shot of a swimming rag. K-Mart, Woolworths, Sears – not ghetto, just functional, budget grandma cute and close. Children are just so small at that age. But she didn't. And I certainly didn't mention this idea. Of course, it's not like there was any great sense of decorum. Even through all the liquor and fake best intentions, the thing knew exactly what I wanted the video for.

I met this liquor soaked and dead witch at a hooker's bar – what everyone calls a hooker's bar – in downstate Illinois. Talked to her awhile, did what I had to do, and came back a few times later. She smelled out my intentions – not a hard thing to figure out given the intimate circumstances – and offered to sell me this tape; this very, like I said before, innocent video tape.

This thing sucked my cock for twenty dollars and offered her cunt for thirty more. I told her when I was going to cum and she slid her mouth away but kept jerking my dick with her hand in about the same rhythm. Which was nice. She had tugged a saggy drugged sucked limp tit out of her tacky whore's black biker blouse – too tight for a mother with fat lumps but, I think somewhere, that's the point. She struggled out bar napkins from her front pocket (black jeans) and handed them to me after I came. She didn't offer to clean up me or the mess on the floor as she was standing by then. We had repaired to one of a few different small rooms in the back of the bar. To do this. Like little washing rooms for laundry – no machines or tubs or dusty sinks or plastic lines stretched across the walls, but that was the basement stink of the place.

It was a terrible place to be. And a terrible mistake all the way around. When first led back there – for only twenty dollars, very quickly – I realized how stupid I was being. This was still hot in the front of my mind as my eyes adjusted to the sudden dark light (the walk back there was nearly pitch black) and she stood there expecting me to – what – suck on her revolting breast or grow hard by its tease. Pet her, force her head down by my palm hard on the top of her rat's nest or hug or just unzip? A charming touch to the room was a small bathroom rug on the floor that she knelt on to undo my pants and blow me. I expect we would have gone somewhere else if I had picked up the offer to fuck her cunt. It had dawned on me that I could be very vulnerable back here and my cock responded more to this than to her far too industrious hands. Spit on her palm. Grabbed my dick. Brushed the tip with her tongue and lifted and licked the underside of the shaft. Looked to see if there was a pre-cum drop. Or syphilis perhaps. Then gulped me up and sucked, exaggerated, hard. I felt my balls tighten and my cock stretch and thicken. I heard her head pop as she checked at the degree of hard-on and tickled the dry piss hole with her fat tasting tongue. Any minute some big biker fuck is going to come up behind me and smash me unconscious. I told her to wait by brushing my hands against her shoulders and plopped out of her sloppy dog mouth. I walked exposed behind her kneeling slump and saw the hideous mop of teased and wired and old combed colored and split hair she wore like it might actually matter to some particularly close drug addict or specific john. Pimp, neighbor, mother, gang. Her and her make-up and that female fucking dug pushed up and hung out and fat and sick. The air and cold spit and flash of my dick as I stumbled around the thing did more for my hard-on than her taffy pull technique and porno tongue would ever know.

  I started to get hard before she even – quickly – shifted back around to face my cock. I wanted to have my back to the wall and my face towards the paper board accordion door. That I then saw was completely shut. And her body in between.

  She said nothing, just opened her mouth and that white girl whore tongue and that ugly female practiced whore's rhythm. Fine. Cunt. I knew then, like I know now, it wasn't the blow-job at all, honey. Thing.

  I wondered if I should reach down and pull her dug. I thought it might be polite. I wondered if I was obligated. I feared if I went anywhere near the sandbag I'd pinch it til she yelled and I knew that would: be a mistake. Cost extra. I came. Her on her knees, moving her head to the side of my thigh and looking away. Like I was an ill child and she was doing her motherly best to help me vomit over a toilet she didn't want to look into.

Thanks. Come back anytime she told me, as she tucked herself together, standing, making my position there and back at the bar obvious. I should just leave.

I walked out towards the dark passageway, less dark now, through the bar, head slightly down and careful not to give anyone the wrong kind of look. The light outside was late afternoon. That was a big fucking mistake. AIDS, VD, a robbery could still happen and any cop could have been anywhere. Never again. Never fucking again. I had lost control. I had put myself in jeopardy for something as ...ugly ...as simple and easy and fucking overpowering as filling some cunt's anything with my dick. I had given up to a weakness inside me. Something above me, prodding and pushing me. Separate. Animal. Like the rest of the dogs sat at the bar. Some fucking connection to something else pulling strings and mapping out blind directions and group dance instructions. Schizophrenic. I knew better and had to be better than the situation which suddenly seemed so important and huge that I'd completely forgotten: what I wanted in the first place. There is no beauty in strength. There's no truth in weakness. There is absolutely no such thing as nature. Not now. Nothing that I belong to anyways.

I knew it wasn't the stench of female. I knew it wasn't some fucking hole or some black stupid drive. I just got in line. It wasn't what I wanted, but it was available.

That ugly pig would always be there. I knew that. And if not her – if, say, she died of an overdose of crystal meth; white biker type mother trash that all her sort seem to obsess over rather than the crack and liquor favored by wasted niggers and junk favored by the spindly city punks, there'll be another cunt – vagina, literally – in exactly the same bar exactly like her any-fucking-where. This I knew with every fucking fiber of my being. Face fucking this particular thing was hardly necessary. Seeing the fucking thing sitting in the bar was just as good – just as necessary, as desired – as seeing her drooping flesh and soaking mother's tongue lapping my dirty smells and cheap cumming heat. Even watching her. Being there where she seeps. Putting myself in that position: It was all too desperate.

Fucking her hollow head made sense there only. Fucking her hollow head with my cock there pushing in and out like a dog made sense only after I gave up to something other than the reality of the bar, to the attraction to the pained caged beast, the thing, in the first place. It was, very simply, very definitely, a bad decision made from a lust that ceased to have definition. My tastes had become excuses, like some mother of a crippled child might label her crowded days and forced plans: spiritual. What I wanted was inconsequential to what I – apparently – had to do or was allowed to do or pushed to do.

Conned; a bait and switch.

And this held true for all my return visits there. I had eliminated the police from the equation by not going into the back bar after that. Even when this thing rubbed my jeaned crotch under the table and tried to start a – what – free hand job, paying hard-on. I'd let her outline and pinch all night if she felt like it. Which she didn't. I didn't get hard. That way. And I'd take her hand away when she tried to pop buttons.

Of course, I paid her. And didn't spend near enough time with her. For the price. I told her I'd be happy to just sit there and talk and find out certain things and she should feel free to go with whoever she felt like if she saw an opportunity. She was hardly pleasant or even accommodating. But to her credit, she knew – after the first time – that I didn't want to talk about my problems or myself and that I didn't believe her talk show white trash tales for the lonely. Father abuse didn't ring true and it was clear to both of us that, although a nice gesture on her part, I was just this very irritating pest worth some easy money if, after being paid, she could get me out quick enough.

I did not want to be this beast's friend. In any way. Even professionally. I didn't want to drink with her and know the name of the bartender or her co-whores or traders. I liked the stories about her daughter. The thing got it after awhile. As she went down the list.

I liked looking in her pinched and wrinkled face and checking the dilated pupils, the whiskey sweat, the unwashed hair and the way words could slur and mash altogether on the way out of her stupidly hung sloppy maw. What she said, I knew and proved, would be of very little consequence.

Her wretched spleen. Her slab liver. And why she had to pee so often.

Her dreams of being better than this, her excuses, and Speed sense.

Her child. Singular.

Her buddies here at the bar. Cash family.

Downtime. Painkillers. Time wasters.

How nice, at least, I was. And then she tried

to sell me on a little more: I had hurt her mouth, I was one of the thickest dicks she had ever had. Just a little more than usual.

Her child was not sacred ground. No hidden secret, no untouchable place that only close friends and better customers can go. No mother clouded pose either. It was very simple. I kept asking and she, lazy as she so quickly was, never felt the urge to make up porno tales. She knew my interest was specific and her answers became genuine, first in an attempt to dissuade me from asking more. I didn't want to know about her fucks and the possible rape scenarios while she was out peddling her flabby cottage cheesed asshole. She got to that by talking about the laundry not being done, and not smoking in the house, the price of Pampers and how quick she had to mend clothes because of their short lifespan as the child doubled in size every damn month. School girl recess rote.

She told me nothing about the father or how the little rat was the best thing in her life. How maybe she felt terrible about what her life had become and the need to get out before it affected the child. Which, of course, was the real reason she kept on. She never even mentioned the poverty angle which, business wise, might have seemed appropriate.

She told me how she liked to swim. How she bought a new bathing suit for the baby and how the baby liked to wear it around the house, baby talking about when they were going to go to the beach again. 'Cause she knew momma liked it there too, the thing could have added for effect, but didn't. The child was sold properly selfish. I understood, but made the usual fucking stupid allowances and comments anyway.

And she told me about the video. And I said I would like to see it. No problem. Price and, yes, there was nothing vulgar about it at all. Lest I get arrested for child pornography as that was hardly my interest. Correct.

The possibility of being primed crossed my mind. There's more you could ask for. More that she or others could provide. Or that video was at her apartment, where other, better, services were available.

There is no baby bald tight cunt in this video. No changing scene, no trace of anything but a large cumbersome and ugly diaper bunched up underneath this little orange flat slick bathing suit. No little three year old ass cheeks sneaking out from behind. Fuck's sake, take the diaper off before you dunk it in the water you mindless inconsiderate slob.

Longish stringy wet then drying hair. Bright big eyes that I can't see the color of. Baby teeth and a wide giggling smile with pale skin and red cheeks, nose and slight chin. High forehead and soft messy but controllable hair – yellow to blonde to brown when wet and tangled. No nose at all sometimes it seems, little darling. Tiny shoulders with straps just barely separate from the top of her chest and neck and arms.

Fucking little Peanuts pail with sand and plastic blue shovelled out into the wet foam. Running into the water with just her tip toes and being led back into the tight arms of her mother. Or holding hands with mom's girlfriend when mom is manning the camera. All chubbiness stretching into skinny girl with baby face stupidity. She doesn't know anything yet. Not anything real.

The poses and fun are for the child. And

they're done with either snapshots and TV memories, or me, in mind.

Both women talk at the child. But there is not one drop of life there. No boyfriends' names mentioned or daddy or questions asked by the child about where they're going later or isn't this better than – say, something else – or is that man going to come later or do you have to work tonight or even a slight blemish or band-aid innocent enough. The mother, the thing, and friend are suitably dumpy, hardly sexy if not uncomfortably shielding their zaftig laziness and there, obviously, for the child. Within reason. I can easily imagine the rank vodka and coffee breath, the hang over wrinkles and aches, the sore arms and jaws. Their last chance lesbianism.

What if they went out and did this video just for me.

As innocent and clean – and unassuming – as it is. What if they took the little darling out with their camera expressly for this sick fuck pervert at the bar.

Was her friend worried about where this sort of thing could lead? Did she plan with someone else to mug me the next time I came to the bar because, obviously, I didn't deserve to exist. Child fucker. Fat jagoff.

Was I so pathetic? Was it just a laugh? Did either whore worry about the implications and how their relationship had changed just because of this little design and their proximity to some prick as fucked up and lonely as this?

Or did it exist, perfectly, just for the memories it promised to serve up. Did it deliver the nice comfort smiles and tough responsibilities when they watched the tape later. Like any other stupid cunt mother looking for her back to be patted or for a quick dip into never was, never will be, wouldn't it be nice chastisement. And has that all changed, all been dirtied, by its sale to me. And by their decision to sell it to me. Are we watching the same thing. Now?

Could she look at the video the same way ever again. Would mother remember me and my interest when she snuggled the child into the swim suit ever again. Will she have to buy a new one. And burn the old one. Would she question her hugs or looks and turn what was just fucking fine before into something altogether ugly now and, definitely, unsafe. Ugly. Perverse. Purchased. Saleable.

Would she remain indifferent. Drugged to the gills where the answer was money: The details just don't read that way. In any way, asshole: Your problems are your own.

That mouth that tasted my dick and walked away from the table we sat at to talk to another possible blow-job for another twenty bucks was filled with more than meat and heat and stink. It was filled with reality and the metal taste of speed and teeth and the bottom line is only reached when someone asks her to sell it. So don't. And it, honestly, didn't exist before that.

Which is what I bought. Perfect.

There are specific ways of looking at this whole circus. Event. Mess. Destruction. My little doll, I think her pig mother told me, was supposed to be four years old. A lovely age for her mother to raise. A perfect time behind that buzzing scowl and drunk splotches and cock breath to go home night after night to. But the video confuses certain truths then. Would a four year old wear diapers?

And this edges what I see. On the video and into that cunt's face that I pissed cum into.

Did she, maliciously, put a big diaper on her child. So I couldn't see that cradled four year old shadow of ass crack. Or did she put it on the child to sell her as even younger. A tease. A safety.

The sound is badly recorded. Still, I don't hear any names being used.

Or did the little darling not learn to live without it yet? Stunted; maybe the mother is unable to teach the little retarded girl, rapidly turning, slowly discovering, every minute of every needle infected puffy bruised arm slow nod day.

Who takes care of it at home. And what is she doing right this minute. Both of them. Dropping off in the middle of a TV blank and the little bored damage soaking into shit on the floor staring at an old worn couch, infomercial, bare lightbulb, torn and taped photograph, works, a boyfriend rubbing his pants and figuring a little teach and pull and lick scream might peel the right way down his spine just now. His cock hard. Getting hard. His finger can help judge the deepness of her age as far as he can get it inside that non-slash yet and those guts that have to sit way too close given that baby squashed size.

Fuck the junkie.
Let's make another baby, nigger.
Fuck only the hole that's legal.
Fucking thing. Can it talk now?
Which is another possibility. Was the youngster filmed at three, perhaps. And the video is older than a year now. Two years old to three years old is a definite distance, she's at least three but four is a possibility: that long hair, her mouth that answers and squeaks clipped baby sentences that

the fucking camera can't quite pick up.
 I know what I want. And what I got. And, so, it's all true. And sitting there in front of me.
 You cheap used whore.
 You bag of slow death and disease.
 And its toddler.
 When you hold your baby girl, do you feel it in your numbing, peeling ageing womb? Your stretch marks? The split between your grotesque vagina and gaping plugged asshole. I know your kind of filth. You are special that way. You have quite a few good years left in you, right? That sub-human romantic phantom pain has to count for some grace, right, you toilet. You are that thing that sits on the end of any cock anytime.
 Does your belly – your seething empty womb – ache with loss or promise when you view your baby rolling and barking and just screaming. Or just playing. Tickling. I want to see how that baby howls. In pain. In real pain. Different pain. And I want to hear her talk baby talk about what it feels like. All to you. At you. And see the effect. The change. The reality and honesty of motherhood. Or of drug abuse. Or of lazy beasts shitting out more beasts under tree stumps in sleepy paying jungles.
 Where's mommy?
 What does dad's dick taste like?
 How do you weigh a gram of coke?
 Do you feel embarrassed without clothes on?
 Do you know what virginity is?
 What happens when ...who made that hurt?
 Who hurt you? Who hurt your bottom?
 Do you hate mommy?

Do you hate it when she leaves? Do you know where she goes?

Do you want to taste something nice?

Do you know what love is?

How about sex? Drugs? Are you having fun at the beach? You like your bright little outfit? Who are you wearing that for? Does it make you feel pretty? Sexy? Do you think mommy is proud of you? Do you like that? Want to make mommy happy?

Do you like shopping at the 7/11 and Woolworths?

Do you get by?

Do you have everything you want?

I like it when you giggle.

This is my favorite part.

Do you know why mommy looks that way? Do you know the chances of you getting those exact same slits and stains at the corners of your mouth and curve of your lips and crows-feet and jowls and deep wrinkles and used and abused junk speed teeth are mighty good? Dear? When I look at your video, I see your mother. And when I see your mother, you, as well.

When I see her just breathe. I see you, honey. Beautiful. Just like you are. A little package of promise and inconvenience and your mother just beating and bubbling over to let herself out of all that is you. Screwing herself deeper into your little receptacle self.

What is good?

What do you like?

What in this material world makes you smile?

What do you remember. And how does it affect you. What did you bring with you.

What would it mean to do exactly as you'd like?
What would that be?
What is sex without love?
What is pornography without humanity ...without some specific, however slight, sense of human connection? Empathy.
What chance have you got? Now? Left?
What is more ...natural... cumming or failure?
How many fingers are you? I'm bad at guessing ages – you have to help me learn. It's important.

"COCK-HUNGRY AND PREGNANT.
This video features a cute, blondish girl who must be about nine months pregnant. It starts off with her masturbating, until her boyfriend comes in and she eagerly sucks his cock. For a brief minute, another guy enters and she sucks both of them. This video has some real hot fucking and sucking action – don't miss it!
85 Minutes."
(The Tiffany Amateur Collection, T-1732)

I have fucked mothers. I know the truth of the universal mother and its stench of biology. I've paid the universal mother ten dollars to cum in its mouth over its cunt. I've fucked its bruised and scarred and small poxed pitted black ass and cleaned its shit off my cock with a crumpled up plastic bag from Walgreens. The stink that still sticks to my moneyed cock and burns my thighs and eyes is the same stink that clings to the yellow grease stains slathered all over their cardboard cages called housing projects.

I like it when the rats open their tiny little brains and squeak: follow your heart.

There are rooms in Cabrini Green that cost $18.00 a month in rent. I hear. Apparently your rent is based on your welfare status and it's understood that whatever the amount, it'll just go unpaid. Understood by the various agencies organised to look after the lots: whose jobs it is to help out the helpless and their money allotments, their gang problems and drug and abortion and AIDS and black on black crimes and babysitting and child abuse and neglect and teen work and education and Sunday BBQ god or neighbor meetings and jobs-for-the-future programs.

How many shitting screaming little black babies can you pile on top of how many fat drunk lazy garbage mouthed mamas? How many chemically shivering sweaty sliding nigger punks can you pile on top of their borrowed rusty bathtubs, broken windows, unused but free condoms and flea beds? How many angry squealing rats can you lock one atop the other until they rip their way outside their tight fucking cages. They gnaw at and eat each other first, don't they?

They say: follow jesus.

Save the children. An equal chance.

Brother, can you spare a dime.

I've seen the caucasian colored flesh split from inside nigger whore's cunts. Inside those blacker than the deepest tar soaked stomach cancer, gristled labia lips spread out sticky pink. Hideous keloidal white flesh stained cunt. Like their palms. And the bottoms of those nail stung feet. The inside of their lower fat rubbery lips. Ugly that way.

I don't know how crowded those rooms get. I don't know how hot they bake when the humid Chicago boiling sun roasts all the barbwire and unpainted rusting metal. All the chicken coop netting and broken locks and splintered cracked wood. How the walls split and warp from crack clouds and steaming drooled body fluids and rank overcooked pork grease.

Then there's some ones that I'd never allow for. Possibly. Maybe. Probably very different from the stereotype I fully intend on believing. The ones that hide. The ones huddled in frightened corners. The ones with even worse luck, perhaps. Probably. But.

They're all the same.

The universal mother exists and protects and breathes inside all of them.

And I like it when it's poor. And lost. And hungry to angry degenerates into frenzied hopelessness. Sometimes accepting and always rotten with stupidity and mental disease and so few options.

Ask it to take its top off completely. Its cheap knock-off sports grey t-shirt. Over its head and crinkled slicked flat unclean hair and above its brutalized skinny dugs. In the front seat of a hardly safe car. And it bursts into tears.

Please help me.

I haven't made anything tonight.

It had to see its bruises.

And it'll take just a minute to forget it completely again and again.

Its child and the bruises it came in here with. They are exactly the same kind – in the same places – I could have given him. That I can make larger and deeper red and blue black and make hurt just a little bit different than the one that's on his skinny boney knee from falling down as he ran into the big black iron doors at toddler school. Or onto the hot dirty concrete. The glass smashed and hidden in old browning grass and mud.

Or the bruises made from his owner's disinterest. Neglect. Impossibilities. Drunken drugged whorish stupor. Or its stress point: My god, woman, don't you see those signs on the buses – don't you know the phone number to call when you just can't take it anymore and it only makes sense to abuse your easily produced brood?

What part of daddy's brain made that?
What part of daddy's dick do you like best?
Now; after you've been with him for awhile?

Do the johns make the same face as daddy did when they squash whatever they have into whatever part of you you're able to sell tonight. Crack hurts your teeth just now, doesn't it? You tell me if you've seen that face before on the one who squats down to shut up your child. Does the child's face register the same as yours. He's got your nose; whose tongue does he have?

In the right circumstances, I find its children attractive. In the proper context. Safe and removed. The context that it so desperately clings to and dreams of and blindly accepts as denied but owed. Its children are revolting product. Parcels of its sickness and disease and laziness.

And it's in those realities that I find it so perfectly attractive: its thin skin ready and lined up to sell like another huge cow on a flat stainless steel floor with a thick brown chain nailed into its hooves.

I like hoping the child will live. I like the idea of scissors being plunged into its spine to kill it, or to help it after an unfortunate accident. When we pray, at the same time, for his little body to stay breathing, for him to just make it. At least. Existing. But it'll learn to regret it. Brain pumping lungs half dead without a spinal connection. Breathing with metal and plastic. Under a brand new waft of crack pipe heat.

She made a big fucking mistake.
She asked for it.
Fucking hoped for this.
It earned it. It deserved it.
This is what it gets. This is nature. This is perfect in something's – someone's – plan. And it has to accept that. Now.

Stupidity can be made into a religion. Just like loss. More and more rats sucking each other's cocks and swollen baby bellies and alcohol bottle ends for that last stale drop, blunts and pipes so hot they can't even hold them anymore.

Those that don't deserve an opinion deserve nature.

Like your mother. Like your absent father.
Your mother who sucks cock on cue.

Some nightmare in flesh full of motherly promise in spirit only squeezes her lumpy fat dugs all over some seventies stoned long cock and heavy packed balls. She moves her bags up to his hairy mouth and pinches, tweaks and twists her pink rubbery nipples. A dirty non-white liquid drips slowly from the udder into the gaping maw of the fool who can barely raise his head to lick, first, then suck. At her teat. At her femalia. Like a baby. Like a nested bird. Like a full grown man growing more drugged dead and malleable. His head falls back onto a pillow while the mother hooker lifts her fleshly sacks up so that the camera can correctly record all her paid worth. Mother's filthy milk can now be wrenched from its bloated weight in great aggressive streams – uncontrollable shotgun lines of warm milk shooting and splotching the wasted supplicant's face, swallowing throat, lapping tongue, sunken chest and everything else – old bed, tacky stickered walls, camera pimp, rented lights and cables – within sickening spitting distance. The leaking and squirting sow has directions to lower her punctured motherhood down to the limp folded cock and to rub and gyrate the sad loose wet mess altogether. Then back up to the sucking dog, down to his chest, now back to his cock which either pig, if they absolutely have to, can work up into a quick hard-on. Unless the drugs are too powerful. Or the money's not enough. Or the woman is just too grotesque by this point. Mix his dead-end cum with her whored milk – just like nature intended.

This lactating beast gets to be fucked again.

It doesn't get its period when it can still produce milk. When the baby, or whoever has enough money or time, stops suckling, her period will – naturally – start up again.

During the seventies, those interested could enjoy film loops of these hookers doing their jobs projected into tight booths usually located in the back of most adult book stores. One could choose from the list at the entrance to the arcade or search over the boxes stapled to the doors of the individual booths. Among all the other peccadillos; Poppin' Mamas meant naked pregnant fucking, Milk Maids would include lactating tits.

Many of the booths also had glory holes

drilled into the sides so that after watching some pig approximating your wife and mother, you could stuff your face with the cock of a stranger, similarly affected, and further approximate the experience of motherhood. Those heterosexuals staunchly masturbating at their easy access or unrealized moans were quickly reduced to their situation as desperate hungry faggots made their intentions suddenly all too clear. Sooner or later everyone – everyone – is on their knees with the taste of someone else's cum on their tongue. The difference between motherhood and fatherhood becomes more than who points the dick. Who owns a dick. Who sucks it with whichever specific part of its body. That special perversion of the – very pure – survival instinct. Instinctual. Inculcated. Needful. Mined.

    There is a desire to see that blood.
    And what is formed from it. Hurt.
    These cunts want the chance to live that life that'll include that little mommy passed fairytale: you too, darling, will start to decompose and bleed and expel and leak and sprout and carry and seep and hate and bloat and push and produce and turn it all loose instead of wrapping it in gauze and chiffon and silly little brutal dreams and wishes. You too, sweetheart, will swallow. It all. And this is how.
    I've got the footage courtesy of these very same talking empty-armed parents. The little bundles of slow motion joy with edited piano strolls and voice overs. The mothers lower their heads or tilt them in shame and memory terror or rest them on their blank outraged and robbed husbands' drooping shoulders. Red neck morons whose dicks smell worse than the rapists and molesters and

murderers, who plugged and burned the little wastes of time and space, massage the same heart strings as the fearsome housewives.

I've got Jacklyn Dowaliby in a wading pool. Black wet hair slicked back and smiling just like a child her age is expected to. Full of herself and her parents' video mirror.

I've got Polly Klaas swinging on a swing. Same smile, same giggle, same small hands and mother's dress. Fuller poofier hair and older than dear Jacklyn.

And Polly's dad hisses "Nightmares do that."

There is no Kiddie Porn in this house. No videos, no mommy pictures of any kind that would show, say, a little darling with a cock pushed up to but not fitting inside her little unlipsticked thin lipped mouth, shoved down her bald plain cunt, half inside a thin stomach entered through a stretched out – quite horrifically unnatural – asshole or the way such a little fist tries to wrap itself barely around a full hard thick cock.

No tears. No screams. No nos. No shaken heads and pouts and balled fists and stamping feet and spurting messy erections and illegality of any kind.

Tell me again. Let's watch this one. How exactly did your boy have his little boy penis severed from his body and how did you find him – what did he look like – when you found him tied to a tree, his pants that you picked out and paid for and admired somewhere else in dirt and his crotch area just completely covered in warm clotted and dried and slowly running blood in that filthy black mud and finger stains.

What about the way you had to see your

baby girl laid out on a morgue slab. And see her head crushed into two essential distinct pieces, just mere dirt and bone leather now – not quite the way you remember it, is it? When you think of her and your plans. All those reasons to spread your fatty legs nine months late and shit out something so dear and unprotected as that was.

Do you blame yourself?

Your husband. Society. The motherfucker (literally) who knows what that flesh of your flesh tastes like better than you and what no sounds like when it is wheezed and barked out in painful unfair squeezes and pumps.

I've got photos of Caroline Hogg smiling like Sarah Harper and I've got shots of Robert Black where you can clearly see his fingers. And I know exactly what all three smiles have in common. All ten fingers and two holes, four holes, six holes. I know it.

And I have come to like the lies best. Because real knowledge – reality – is a celebration of exactly what a mess it is that you've made. And the wreck that you prop up and try to hide behind face paint and motherly understood clichés are just about picture perfect. Because they're lazy like you. Like you are now, fat and spent and sucked out dry and like you were, when you let someone – anyone – snatch your little reason to live, your little primped personality, up off her bike and stuff it into the back seat of his car (Brian Dugan), van (Robert Black), and fuck the life (literally) out of it.

I've shared polaroids given to me by a paedophile with a taste for his sister's kids. I've seen them smiling as they sat on his lap, snapped by the sister for her brother. And I've seen shots of the same kids naked and smiling. Taken by the paedophile.

He told me he masturbated with the shots that he talked the children – two very little girls – into posing for. He never fucked them. Though he desperately wanted to. Especially the chubbier one. And he never touched them except to help them into their freshly picked underwear.

Your DNA leaves its mark on a licked envelope or inside a bruise or onto an underwear stain called, briefly, Repressed Memory Syndrome. They can pull your mark from a never rotting never fresh swabbed out rape hole.

You were designed this way. You have little choice that's not either a limbic mistake or genetic truism; socialization just fucks up what little will you hope for. Your snail's trail proves it.

That little baby will grow up and remember those photos you took under the guise of love and innocence, one day when it seems most appropriate and convenient to her new lifestyle choice.

Gym coaches who watch their freshman Highschool boys' classes take their showers.

A screaming red faced in the dark fat father follows his sixteen year old runaway daughter into a large enclosed vacant parking lot. Pulls out his cock. Wraps around a photo he has of his child when she was young and safe and his to do absolutely anything with. Works the photo into his fist, crinkling and ripping, as he jerks his cock with its sharp plastic and paper cuts. Quickly. He runs up to his daughter, his palm working up his cum around and inside the baby fresh smile photo: DON'T TELL. DON'T TELL. I'LL FUCKING KILL YOU IF YOU TELL.

He fucked her mother to produce exactly

what he had. To produce exactly this. His screaming mad confused DNA.

Why, exactly, do women disgust you so much? Away from teenage, pre-menopausal and just post-sag. These cunts bleed, these cunts stink, these cunts pick and yeast and fart and spew and discharge. Veins and hair and that thick clown make-up that somehow has become acceptable: Tell me about honesty, about love and respect and soul and what new spirituality you fell into this week, you great fat sow; now that that wrinkle cream has seeped so deep into your craters and divots that your crows' feet have turned into full personalities of their own.

Skank. Vagina. Beaten motherly hog lying on a sheet covered uncomfy metal table waiting, begging, now, for a two day old C-section and some drugs because those gift given ribs and pit hole just aren't moving quick or far enough apart yet.

You want some painkillers?

You want some comfort.

You want to scratch up flesh and hold on to the edge of the table. You remember when you took those Gym-mat classes and you could wrap those skinny legs and proper thighs back behind your never blonde haired smiling cheek puffed face. So much unlike the greasy horse you've turned into now. Who'd want to fuck anything about you, mother?

The lights work perfectly with the make-up. All those careful accents.

The prostitute lies on her back on a cheap studio bed and rubs and dips in her puffed dry birth-hole with a cream-colored five and dime brand vibrator. Ratty cheap yellow hair thin over black roots pinned and spilled all atop her squashed ape-ish hispanic brown face. Slippery lips, pimples, bumps, half mast stupidity and old zit pocks. Her bloated cancerous belly is huge with a creature, probably nine months along, short on promise and worth: what kind of little shitting mewling animal could this half human barn produce and what will it offer the world after it's slit from an ugly sucking and fucking and, obviously, dirt poor whore's slimy pit?

     You wanna suck off seven guys in a row and let us film it? What do you need the money for? Diapers, drink, rent, groceries, Advil, crack, heroin, the virgin mary, your five other piglets? How's the hot box walk-up? Are the lines at Welfare too difficult to manage with all the baby carriages and playing and screaming for attention? Do you even know the fucking father still? That hump that spilled his waste into you and created the rest of your life in a half-minute jerk off toilet flush. What are the chances that he'll beat you, and the kidling into a daily pulp, if he still lives with you a couple months from now? Just like all the other drunk meat packing mexicans and niggers you've ever been allowed out for.

     She puts down the vibrator and lowers her heavy head towards her monster size sickness. She licks at her swollen mother tits. Thick brown nipples made prune knotted and twisted from glowing motherhood. Pierced nose; tattoos on her hand – gang or prison style. More tattoos will become visible as the video progresses. As she performs doggy style fucks, the faded blue pick marks on her back and flabby ass will become clearer. As she gets plowed into, on her acne'd flat back, the permanent stains around her ankle and wrist show themselves. How could this cheap stupid rat ever feel so committed about anything. How fucking stupid could this ghetto sludge be. How perfect. How she doesn't have a clue, never had a chance; open wide and hope it doesn't hurt. Have something to eat. Smile. Bark. Roll-over. Spread.

Her pubics – that brown mat of rat hair and Brillo wire, streaks across her pregnant pigness and scatters around her pin pushed navel. It screams down to her puffed out asshole and vines up her pitted thighs and ass-cheeks. Five different men fuck her various cunts. Two return for more at later points. Some lick at her birth deformed vagina through her sweaty hair patch. So close to birth. She gets fucked and reamed and dug into: she lies there dumb and bored and listens to her hair grow. She stares up at the ceiling, she performs porn talk and takes loud direction from the crew assembled around her motel throne.

She seems particularly taken with one greasy off-white but dark middle-ager:

The director, off camera, tells her to guess the fucker's nationality.

She tweaks his black nipples and scoots her kneeling pregnant farm disease closer to his body. He'll have to jump off the bed to get his jeans and socks off but for now, only shirtless and kneeling like he doesn't understand the job at hand, he smiles and waits. With her in her tight stretched out red thin teddy clearly not designed for pregnant cows and attempting to dog perform lust, the squat mama slithers: Puerto Rican?

"Everyone says that", he smiles again and lets her rub his slick chest.

Italian?

"No."

Mexican? What!?

"Black and Portuguese."

The crowd off camera laughs. Throughout the entire hour and a half they can be heard talking amongst themselves while the director only occasionally gives instructions above the din:

"Yeah. Yeah. Yeah."

"Use it like a paintbrush."

The phone rings off camera, jokes are told, no one is interested. Including the dogs that mount the motherly holes and baby to be. All seven scenes end with the near or proper latinos jerking themselves off and aiming their cum at the fluid tight belly, tits or chicken skin face. All seem to have problems keeping or getting hard-ons. The beast herself performs only when necessary. But she knows that the demon loafing cocks have to be milked for the scene to change and the meat of the hard day's work to end.

The half-caste puts on a rubber and explains that it's because he doesn't want to irritate his dick which has a little cut on it.

The pig asks him: Don't take a long time.

Like the others. Please. This momma sucks cock, gets tossed around to switch hole after hole and lets the cum that collects on her various lumps seep into her splotchy skin rather than wiping it off. She slurps some cum off of herself and opens her mouth for the facials. She rolls about the creaky bed with all the grace of a walrus stuck in a crag. And doesn't look to understand that the pigholes she offers aren't only female. Here, it isn't defined only by male lust. By nature what – she possesses by simple dint of gender and the luck that comes with it. The rote games she has learned to play. She splits and opens, offers and pushes and glides and accommodates the foreign matter collecting in her cunt and across her abused chest and hairy face. Just like any other marketed cunt. But the vacant defensive banter, the unhealthy slow draws of breath, and stumbling yellowy eyes, the used and re-sold bargain basement femalia, all sell something else. Or something extra. And this little slice of her life becomes more important, more real, than anything the pig actually lives, or exists, through. She is caged. Her mistakes have been captured and displayed. This document – the video and the sale of it; the available marketability – becomes the special event. The real thing. She just dies sooner or later. Her lack of success. The child's head so close to the cocks pushing again and again through her cunt. Her wretchedness. Her low place in line. Her obscene deformity. And the truth that allows prostitutes and all mothers everywhere the possibility of slowly destroying sexy little rat babies by shackling them to ghettos and sexual abuse. Just like this, what money was invented for.

There is no fascination. There is no search for the secrets that women possess. There is no truth to be gleaned from sticking your finger into a cunt, your dick into a mouth or fist in an asshole.

This pregnant mess, this female list of horrors, was here full of cum and quim and lack of sense before you sat down on your couch to watch its pain with your VCR. There is nothing new to be learned about varicose veins, afterbirth or thick black worm fat scars that stretch from asshole to cunt and never ever heal. There is nothing new about implosion or old age. Nothing special or interesting about wilted flesh and chemical changes that cause, conveniently, any newly trade-branded form of depression. Or confused excuses.

There is no fixation.

You didn't see your mother's red rag or douche bag and not forget it. The women you took a bath for, the babysitter in the seventies' tight worn jeans and tube titted top doesn't mean the same as the greasy black whore you pay to stick crack pipes up your ass.

There is no mystery. There are no secrets. You want gospel truth and you want to name it Nature and Mother? You want reason and balance, you need cause and effect? Extra is what you're looking for. What you pulled off the shelf and took home. Extra is specific and personal.

Your mother is a disease. Rotting away and clinging hard to what's there of you.

You get this information in drips as you get older. She was a whore. She ran away from home when she was just a teen and ended up married young. You have a half-sister or two somewhere downstate. When you're old enough to know where to go you put two and two together: you understand where mom ended up and what part of the city gave birth to specific parts of your personality. And mom's. And the sense mom had available to her all her troubled life. That she only needed a price.

That's where all the strip clubs were, back then, wasn't it?

That guy sounds like a pimp.

Have another gin and tonic, souse.

You were so lucky to meet a guy like dad.

Where did you meet him?

Where did you meet a hump like him? A trick, a john, a niggerish dick boy and his cheap needs and your cheaper offers.

How much did last night's cum cost you?

What kind of whore were you?

Who did you fuck when you were pregnant and for how much? Were you able to lift your packed and plugged and whinnying weight around with the same stupid slow clumsiness that that fucking hispanic pile does, when she falls face flat and sells her expanding hole to whatever dog stands behind her?

Can your little baby feel that cock?

And those strange tongues and fingers and intentions?

This pig found herself this way. This pig didn't choose this for herself. This pig nailed herself to that bed and those cocks and those cameras and that consuming churning seething belly like a blind dog sniffs a pile of shit searching for just a bit of non-toxic sustenance. You don't shit into toilets like her. Some germ might crawl up your ass. You stand away and piss into it. You stand well away and aim your cock like a paintbrush. You aim for the mouth, the tits, the embryo, the dirty water that is made for your waste. And when you miss, you're just another privately minded slob. This is a bad neighborhood and you knew the toilet was going to be a pigsty when you entered. You zip up and walk out. Let the next pig flush. Let the pig swallow if she wants the right amount on her paycheck.

The customer creates the interest.

If it wasn't pregnant it would have nothing to sell.

The real beauty of motherhood.

You wanna make $200.00?

What else do you have to offer?

Sometimes you just have to do what you're told.

Darling; are you pro-choice? Do you feel you have the right to make decisions about what you can do or not do with your body? Do you think women can be trusted to make the right decisions? Do you think they can come up with the right answers?

And you? Did you make the right choice? Did you fucking plan this? Did you work it all out beforehand? Are you, at least, happy with this situation?

Do you possibly want this?

Forever? For the rest of your life? Do you still hope all of this will work out?

Did you even have a fucking choice?

Did little baby make a mistake? And are you tied to this now? Did you miss your appointments at the doctor? Do you think that spearing that little worm inside you on the end of a coat-hanger or sucking it down the wrong end of a vacuum tube could be murder? Or is that fucking tiny parasite slowly murdering you – steadily constantly sucking off of everything you were and had. Reducing every inch of your life in mind bleeding never ending bits and pieces.

Was it your choice? You? What part of you? When you closed your cunt around some hard-on and let it spit? When you hoped that he pulled out in time, wore a rubber, cummed on your asshole and not in your cunt, that he wouldn't come back and do it all again by leaving his deposit warming up and grabbing and affixing itself to the walls of filth inside you.

Is that what you spread for? Some fun? That giggle that was just waiting to be let out?

I don't believe any of you. I do believe that the entire act – your whole history – is defined by watching your plans whittled away by your lack of choices. Your options are simple. Your decisions are drooled excuses. You can't ever catch up.

You should have had an abortion.
You look sick this way.
You should have had your legs fused shut.
You should have a few more brain cells.
You should have been born male.
You shouldn't have had that cigarette, one last drink, that condom should've been checked under a better light. You shouldn't have believed in love, lust or second chances.

You should have let the doctor pull the plug when it came out too soon and fit in the palm of his hand.

You should have run away.
You should have thought a little harder.
You shouldn't talk like that.
You shouldn't think those things – it'll only make things worse. You just have to take one day at a time. Now. You just have to get through all of this.

You wanna make some extra money?
You need something.
You know that, at least.
You do need some money – for all of this. For everything you need to get now. And maybe for something you want. Maybe for something that you wanted once and now need to just feel whole again. Something you need more of.

You deserve it.
You just gotta.
You wanna make some money?
It's your decision.
You let me know. I got five guys – two of them want to go twice, so a total of seven and

they want to feed your pregnant face with their good clean cum. Just like you've done before.

The fucking baby won't know.

There's an audience out there who likes to look at your bloated busting pig meat and the holes you continue to offer.

Would you like to try?

Your choice.

You can turn a bad thing – well, not that that's bad, right, I mean, it's a wonderful thing, it's just that times are hard now ...you can turn a rough situation to your benefit.

No one would want to pay you extra if we weren't paying for two.

Now is important. Right now. This minute. These next few days will be better than the last few – and a baby is all future, isn't it? That's what's important.

Let me help you.

Let us help you.

Let us help both of you.

It's your choice. Your noisy mind. It's all yours to sell.

I think it must be drugs. Every time I see one of you beasts moving so slowly, so sickly, I can't imagine you believe in what you've done.

Am I wrong to have given you the benefit of the doubt?

Reach over. Put your head down. Mother. Bite that soft baby head. Let your teeth peel into that soft as shit never healing baby bendable head. Squash it. Knock it down stairs. Suffocate it. With your not inconsiderable weight. Pinch its tiny nose before it's too late. Pound its chest – just once, you don't have to do it too hard, its heart will burst easily, it's a very fragile sickness. Throw it against the wall or shake it quickly up and down, ghetto sludge style. Make it quit screaming. Quit sucking you dry.

Put it in the back of your car and drive it into the water. Lock them in their baby seats. Fill those fresh lungs with heavy bleeding and rupturing black water full of parasites and filth and disease. Rape their small bodies with frightened death.

Mop the floor with her face and shrinking cries. Feed her her feces that she wiped all over the refrigerator in the grip of a frenzied seven year old mental breakdown. Put her down on the bed like a retard; she having fallen unconscious after being raped repeatedly over days – using a toothbrush and a hairbrush inside her little flowered and dead and morgue creamed body. Make the children stop bullying you into being something you're not.

Feed them poison. Tear up their tight fleshed bodies with grease from the pans on the stove, finger fuck whatever hole offends – or excites – you most.

Make them swallow glass shards and vomit blood and spit tears.

Funnel in bleach.

Film their injected quaking bodies and sell the one and only video to a pervert you heard about: who stays at home and masturbates – only masturbates – to films that hurt children and promises more. Let him fund your crimes. Let him plant that germ for more crimes, longer lengths, better ideas.

Inject your body with heroin and crack and shit the baby out shivering and silent screaming and frying and film it like some yuppie in hospital blue fake smiles would. Let's see it bathed in your sick blood flopping around like an unhooked suffocating fish too terrified and bone soft to audibly bark. Slide it across the floor. Dirty; cut by splinters and your own long painted nigger nails. For a camera close-up.

Defecate. Shit. Pinch and strain. Let your unhealthy AIDS crack porcelain bleeding squirting bodily waste burn its flesh. Let nature be your guide. Celebrate all that is human. Whatever disease you've let crawl into your black chewing and spewing body, whatever has attached itself inside your sewer female hole for as long as that thing you made tumbled and recoiled and suckled dry nothing dust.

Let me convince you. Hold the baby down and let it expire. Let it die by not touching it. Let's see what happens. Let that five pound malformed bag collapse and implode and fight its handful of fight to stay alive as if it knows absolutely nothing else. Let its tiny little body eat itself. Its snap and sinew, its baby fat and cold brain. That is nature. That's nature like the idea was sold to you. See if those paper thin chicken skinned giblets blend and fuse and grow and create anything worthwhile. Or if it just shakes and coughs up blood bubbles and nothing at all in its – only shadow staring – eyeless brain.

What did you want?
What did it get from you?

"**Q: What about fisting?**
Jamie Gillis: Okay for your personal collection, but unsellable to a distributor."
(PERVERT CUM LAUDE, Chuck Farnham, *The Nose*, #24, September, October 1994)

"The prosecutor says the defendant and Karla took turns taping each other violating the girls. During one disturbing sequence, Bernardo pretends he's directing a pornographic movie and makes his wife and Kristen dress up in school uniforms, the court was told."
(VIDEO MONSTER, *The Star*, June 6, 1995)

"'You watched the (sex) tape on other occasions with Mr. Bernardo, didn't you, Miss Homolka?'
 'No, I didn't; you're very wrong,' Karla replied.
 'You watched it, and you enjoyed it, and you got a big laugh out of it because it's part of the kinky sex you were into,' said Rosen.
 'That's a lie,' Karla shot back."
(DEADLY INNOCENCE, Scott Burnside and Alan Cairns, Warner Books, 1995)

"Among the disorders Bernardo may suffer from, according to Hucker: paraphilia (sexual deviation), sexual sadism, voyeurism, hebephilia (attraction to pubescent or adolescent females), toucheurism (grabbing of unsuspecting women), coprophilia (deriving sexual excitement from feces), alcohol abuse and narcissistic personality disorder. Still, Hucker wrote, 'there is nothing I have seen in the evidence so far available that Mr. Bernardo has or has had a major illness of a psychotic type, i.e. he is fully in touch with reality.'"
(BERNARDO: THE UNTOLD STORY, Joe Chidley, Maclean's, September 11, 1995)

1.   *Paris Match*, #2444, 28 Mars 1996.

2. FEAR GRIPS TEXAS TOWN AFTER GIRL'S ABDUCTION, *Chicago Tribune*, January 16, 1996.
9-year-old grabbed while playing, it is her family's second kidnapping.

FOUR

"Each man was given 30 minutes in the cubicle, and I would try and prolong the time in an effort to lessen the number I had to serve, even to lessen the number by one. At first, I got away with this, but later on I was too exhausted to do anything but lie still like the dead with my face turned to the wall, avoiding his stare."
(Yi Okpun, TAKEN AWAY AT TWELVE, TRUE STORIES OF THE KOREAN COMFORT WOMEN, Edited by Keith Howard, Cassell, 1995)

"One man, although drunk, stayed inside me his whole allotted hour. It was unbearable – but I had to bear it."
(Madam X, THE COMFORT WOMEN, George Hicks, Souvenir Press, 1995)

"The girls might smile for no reason, or perhaps they smiled at the prospect of earning 500 baht for an hour's work instead of 70 baht for a day hauling cement on a building site in 90-degree weather. That's a little over two dollars a day but for most of them, that was the only alternative."
(Rory O'Merry, MY WIFE IN BANGKOK, Asia Press, 1990)

"In 1984, five young girls who had been imprisoned in a Thai brothel were burned to death in a fire. Later it was revealed why they'd never had a chance: They had been chained to their beds."
(David Hechler, CHILD SEX TOURISM, Appendix to BATMAN: THE ULTIMATE EVIL, Andrew Vachss, Warner Books, 1995)

"A hierarchy of jobs existed on Patpong. Working in a blow-job bar, like Dang, or performing in Fucking Shows was at the bottom."
(Cleo Odzer, PATPONG SISTERS, Blue Moon Books, 1994)

"'I don't have any money. I'm pregnant. I'll be leaving work. I need the money.' I went with him. He wanted to do things to me that I didn't like, such as three holes. He said he would pay me for that."
(Madelin, LET THE GOOD TIMES ROLL, Saundra Pollock Sturdevant and Brenda Stoltzfus, The New Press, 1992)

"If I were a man, I'd never entice a kid into working the streets, even if she were low on money and bumming rides. I'm starting to hate men except for fatherly fantasy figures who are gentle, comforting, and couldn't possibly have real penises."
(RUNAWAY: DIARY OF A STREET KID, Evelyn Lau, Coach House Press, 1995)

"While mizu shobai women provide a service judged to be socially legitimate, the legitimacy

of the service extends only to the men seeking the service, not to the women servicing the men, who are seen as somehow transgressing their very nature by being sexualized, even in talk, by males. The woman's position then becomes one of degradation – she is the slave."
(Anne Allison, NIGHTWORK, The University Of Chicago Press, 1994)

"It really sucks when you have a 'flashback' onstage. Once some guy spat a mouthful of beer in my face – he was this close – and it reminded me of when I was 15 and being raped, and the guy came in my face."
(Kathleen Hanna, ANGRY WOMEN IN ROCK, Andrea Juno, Juno Books, 1996)

"Sometimes I ponder the idea that hundreds of thousands, perhaps even millions of men (even some women) have masturbated while looking at images of me. I wonder what effect this might have had on my life on a metaphysical level. Perhaps I might have felt it physically. I don't know for sure, but I like to think that my life has been enriched by it."
(Annie Sprinkle, POST PORN MODERNIST, Art Unlimited, 1991)

"Ms. Fox, by any objective judgement, is out of proportion. Her small body, well under average height for a woman, is dominated by a secondary sexual characteristic gone mad, a huge pair of breasts (requiring, apparently, a 38DD bra cup, whatever that may be) which constitutes a constant reminder of her

biological role. Ms. Fox can never know the freedom of going without a bra, without straps and painful bits that dig into her flesh – except, of course, when she is in front of the camera. Her chest relegates her to the position of the crudest of sex objects, one so lacking in subtlety that it is not hard to conjecture that her 'fans' are characterized by the immaturity and functional nature of their sexual response."
(Joan Smith, MISOGYNIES: REFLECTIONS ON MYTHS AND MALICE, Fawcett Columbine, 1989)

"There is a lot wider variation in men's conscious attitudes toward pornography than there is in their sexual responses to it."
(Catharine A. MacKinnon, ONLY WORDS, Harvard, 1993)

"We are recognized only as the discourse of a pimp."
(Andrea Dworkin, PORNOGRAPHY HAPPENS TO WOMEN, THE PRICE WE PAY, Laura Lederer & Richard Delgado, eds., Hill And Wang, 1995)

"I took them into their yard behind some shrubs and pulled down the front of my shorts (I wore no underwear on these trips). I said, 'Anyone want to touch it?' The 4-year-old did and said, 'Yep – it's real!' They all laughed, and the 4-year-old and two of the 9-year-olds agreed to meet me at a vacant field nearby that evening so I could do it again and show them some tricks (making it 'bigger', 'bouncing' it without touching it, and making stuff come out), and I might even teach them

how to do it, but they never showed.
      That was the last time I ever flashed a kid. One had touched me, and gave me a better feeling than just showing myself. I now wanted to be touched, not seen."
(Westley Allan Dodd, personal diary, 1976)

"New Orleans Style! Come along with GM VIDEO for a Close in depth Look at All the Action, we mean Action! This Video is so jam Packed with TITS & ASS you won't believe it! Our roving cameras were in the crowds catching all those Beautiful Girls Flashing T&A and BUSH! It's just like you were there. All Spontaneous Action! Don't miss Vol 2 thru 4."
(#170 MARDI GRAS '95 Vol #1 of 4; 2 hrs. Hard R.)

"What a Fucking Hoot! All on Video, GM Style! We topped last year with More Tits. More Bush. More Close Ups. More Nasty Stuff! All Spontaneous, no Staged Crap! Every Size Tits & Ass You could ever wish for! Each Volume Always contains something UnXpected? Don't Miss Vol 2 & 3."
(#184 MARDI GRAS '96 Vol 1 of 3; 90min. X.)

"Unlike many other Videos of Sturgis we didn't spend a lot of time filming all the Harleys. Just all the Girls Flashing their Tits, Ass and Bush! Wild and Crazzy. GM invaded the Camp Sites and RV Parks for a behind the scenes look! Even a Nude Wedding! Don't miss all the Biker Chicks!"
(#177 BIKE WEEK T&A, STURGIS 1995; 110min. Hard R.)

"He's amazing! They call him 'Ugly George, The Professor of Seduction' and 'America's Crude Dude' but if results are what counts, we all have a lot to learn from this funny looking guy with a video camera under his arm! WATCH HIM WORK HIS MAGIC ON INNOCENT YOUNG GIRLS! Every woman wants to show herself, to 'flash her goodies' and delight as she exposes her bouncing breasts and pouting pussy for a man to lust after, admire and worship! But how do you get a girl to 'give in', to surrender to those inner needs and desires? GEORGE CAN SHOW YOU HOW TO GET THEIR CLOTHES OFF ...ANYWHERE! His technique is failproof! He stops strange, beautiful girls on the street ...starts an innocent conversation ...and before you know it, he is chatting and charming them right out of their moist panties ...sometimes in the closest alley or doorway available!

Watch 'Ugly George' do it and then 'go and do likewise' yourself! You'll learn every clever trick, every subtle persuasion device he's taken years to perfect ...and you'll lead a richer, sexier life for it too!"
(ELECTRIC BLUE SPECIAL: UGLY GEORGE, Kenyon Video, 1982, 60 minutes)

"Deep within the concrete canyons of New York City there lurks and thrives a personality so bizarre, so strange, so totally off the wall, that the world knows him only as Ugly George. George is a specialist – a specialist at accosting young, unsuspecting girls as they go about what would have been their everyday business. And what exactly is George after from all these heavy hootered honeys? Their bods, of course! So turning on his ever present video camera, he coaxes and cajoles these unsuspecting damsels into doorway, alley, and even into his private 'Polish Penthouse' for a time they'll never forget and none regret.

So strap yourself in, grab ahold of your 'pencils' (as George himself would put it) and get ready for one of the strangest journeys you'll ever experience – a Totally Unrehearsed, Triple X Rated journey of amateur exuberance and dynamic proportions.

Plus, this video features GRETCHEN, a one-in-a-million find who may just be the World's Largest Busted Woman, in a brain melting bosom love bout with the ugly one himself. Rated XXX."

(TNT TITALATORS: THE BIG BUSTED GIRLS OF UGLY GEORGE, Big Top Video, 1985, 60 minutes)

"A frank, humorous, and provocative documentary about what some men really think of women. Produced by award- winning filmmakers Lucy Winer and Paula de Koenigsberg, RATE IT X is an eye-opening excursion into sexual values in America today.

Men from all walks of life are interviewed – like Ugly George, the cable TV star whose 'gimmick' is to ask women to take off their clothes on camera. There's a baker who creates 'bikini cakes', a lingerie advertising man, a group of retired war veterans, and even a funeral director who shows caskets designed to appeal to men (blue) and women (pink)! It's funny, feisty, and fresh – a new look at an old problem, produced by women with a sense of humor."

(RATE IT X, International Video Entertainment, Inc., 1985, 95 minutes)

That cunt crawled around like a roach. Like a flattened roach looking for somewhere hot to hide; frantic like someone turned the light on too fast.
    On all fours, legs up tight and fixed and arms stretched down straight and fast; cunt looking for some dick. From dick to dick to dick.
    Your wife has been raped.
    What you owned has been stolen. What you bought belongs to someone else.
    She was stuck like a caged farmpig. In her small studio apartment working to pay her bills and do what little she liked. What she was owed.
    What we know – and you don't want to hear this, but you do need to know – is that she was attacked by more than just one man. A group of men.
    You are one dumb cunt.
    You are one disgusting fucking pig: all covered in blood and cum and wanting more.
    What kind of pig would do that?
    You want to know how we know it was a gang that attacked her? That it was more than just some single horny burning nigger following her home from buying whatever it was she needed at whatever unsafe time of night?
    She was a breathing cum towel. She was covered in beer and beer swilled sweat and beer pissed cum.
    You think she deserved better? Because she wanted something else? Because she wanted a break? Just because she didn't want that?
    We know because of the cuts and scrapes

and scratches of all different lengths and degrees that cover her body leading and coming all different ways. Fingernail slices and teeth scar bites and paper cuts and forced squeezed bruises that spread and bleed damage inside. We also know because of her hysteria just before she fell into shock. She was screaming and hallucinating and biting the air. She was lashing out at the technicians, the cops and the medics who were pawing at her and sticking needles and drugs into her. She was frothing about hands and cocks and AIDS and heat and stink and all about her head blacking out being forced under water.

There were foot prints made of blood and grease and smeared with shit and beer.

Crumbled up cardboard that they used to scrape the muddy mess from their shoes and bodies, that was maybe used as a gag or some form of tampon to stop the heavy flow of hemorrhage.

There'll be a full cup of cum inside her.

She'll have to get an AIDS test. And tests for other sexually transmitted diseases. Syphilis is particulary virulent lately. Crabs, herpes, counselling, prozac, morphine.

She's in pretty bad shape.

Why didn't she just chomp off one of those dicks shoved into her bright bawling mouth? They used every hole she has, had: you just know that. Why didn't she just bite down hard.

It's the survival instinct. It's the strongest of all. It must have made sense to her, at the time, to just get to the next moment where hopefully the pain and evil and unfairness and threat and fear would stop.

She sucked when she was told to suck. To

swallow that load you cunt. She didn't want to die all the way.

She'll have to deal with driving thoughts of suicide now. Ironically. She won't be able to take this. Anymore. She'll keep hearing. And saying.

She'll suffer flashbacks and brain lesions and have to fit all she knows about inequity and worth into her new life. Her fucking survival instinct will want to suck up all that cruelty and come up with something special; much more special than what worked before.

That gun that got rammed up inside of her gave her life.

Do you know what you want, whore?

You gotta know what you want in this life.

What do you want most of all?

She must have been fed that gun. That's what happens in a real gang bang. Someone showed her how that steel and power felt cold and hot inside that lame endorphin rushed unnumbed body. Wake up, honey, everything can come crushing down right up from the insides of your skull.

Do you have any friends who can come take care of you?

Treat you right?

They held her down with their fists and dog shit shoes: I don't know if they planned it all out beforehand; if anyone was wearing steeltoed boots or meat packing shitkickers.

Just hold your head there while I fuck it. Hold her head straight while I fuck it like a garbage hole in the dirt. And the rapists were hard from her fear. And from her animal scratched nakedness. He liked the way her tits looked. Firm and not so young and a healthy untouched by a real man cunt, salad stomach not unlike some of the stuff on lighted display but not for sale everywhere else. He got full and rushed from her crying and weak womanly helplessness. Her struggling; weak and pathetic and perfect.

She can be taught classes in self-defense. She can take therapy where she'll be encouraged to cut a rubber dildo in half.

She can wear her damage as a call to arms.
She can never drink alone again.

Her chances for motherhood are well fucking slim. Depending on how old she was, she might have been fucking menopausal for all I know.

How close to pornography did she look when sucking off any other member of the gang. Did anyone fuck her ass and cunt at the same time; cum on her belly or, as is the case when no camera is present: straight down inside its throat or shot up into its womb.

All the blood and cum mixing with her guts and ovum and stink forming a new rat biology out of such ugly natural aggression.

Imagine her next want of cock. Of cunt, of flesh, of comfort or escape or pity.

Her next drink of water from a stainless steel fountain.

Her next hug or good old fashioned cry.

I have this idea.

I'd like to take this child – at times, a girl seems best and at others; I'd like a weepy little boy. For some reason a boy would be much easier to break, I think.

I'd like to keep a child in a box. For as long as it took. Barely feed it. Fuck it always, in all different sexy ways – as one's tastes change in terms of what pornography seems appropriate for whatever sense of proxy is needed whenever. And slowly convince the child to commit suicide.

Convince might not be the right word. I guess I'd like the idea to come from inside the child – not from me talking it into it.

But imagine that: how long would it take. What would the defining moment be?

Like a test in a concentration camp.

Or fucking your wife with the barrel of a gun and about five or six hung cocks – or a very small penis for that matter; in fact, I think short stubby greasy cocks would be best provided there's a coke bottle or Tanqueray, or a chair leg around as well, or half a rubber dildo even – until she just can't take it any longer.

Like ten or so years after she pulls herself up from her nightmares and casts and tries to dance naked in a peep show booth or upmarket strip bar. Sucks a gun off with her finger at the trigger inside the women's bathroom where some of the more liberated or uncaring sisters take quick cash johns for the same kind of non-metallic tasting tongue job.

There's a certain sense of forgiveness that bothers me. If you've ever been around certain streets in New Orleans during Mardi-Gras you'll see obnoxious amounts of flesh. Most likely, it'll be females of all ages, though not really children, pulling down their tops and lifting up their bras and wriggling out tits of all shapes and sizes and deformations.

Some of these women pretend they're flashing their body parts for cheap shiny beads, sexual identification or just plain lazy drunkenness. No matter how ugly, or typically un-pretty, they know the crowd wants to see it. Every slob is in *Playboy*, every beast no longer suffers the horrors and hurt of lookism.

And the crowds go crazy. Some balconies are dedicated to this event and the strip clubs pay their strippers to play along.

Hands – usually a fair amount of black ones – reach out to cup or grab or often pinch the breasts that are flashed and then covered up, or attempted to be, almost immediately. The men hoot and yee-haw and beg and barter and memorize.

Film crews and camcorder jagoffs offer nicer beads and even cash or just the proper sort of attention. They often ask for pink shots, or for the girls to bounce up and down and jiggle or even encourage them to perform blow-jobs or lesbian licks and kisses with their partners.

The video tapes are then sold in regular adult video stores. The ones that feature girls are sold to heterosexual men as "soft-core". The videos that feature men flashing and tugging at their cocks are sold and marketed to gay men as camp and safe and understood.

But aside from the male audience, what the events, and more so, the tapes, have in common is the sense of acceptance and accommodation. Whatever the girls or men get out of the act itself is up to them. Not all men, I suppose, are dogs looking for cunt just as all the women with their tits out and cunts spread are Freudian messes who'll either hate themselves later or work up a new-age excuse of liberation and catharsis and female empowerment. All is fun is a fine excuse. What is important and shared is the fact that so many of the women are hideously ugly.

Great big scars on their fat bellies. Fleshy misshapen nipples and cellulite. Stupid straps and fastens that hide bulges and badly done tattoos and sloth are struggled clumsily out of and snapped open to let all sorts of sicknesses blubber out.

A woman in a wheelchair; its thick heavy flabby jugs flopped atop her protruding bunched up lap forever belly, lifts her tent large overwashed t-shirt up to thunderous applause.

A mother and daughter – wearing home painted shirts that advertise their willingness to flash – display; on the daughter, skinny boned flattened sucked out dry white trash flesh bags limped and hung like wrinkled scars while the mother displays a belly swollen out far below her high pants line and small but equally damaged dust filled waste breasts.

Mastectomy scars and fake hard tits that couldn't possibly have been done purely for someone else's viewing pleasure.

Cancer lumps waiting to happen, for sucking, for mothering, for exhibit and sale and obsession.

And there's the demure attempts, or equally blatant as the case may be, of even the younger just-college kids who've made their reputations on the size of their sweaters and t-shirts that, once exposed, quickly try to hide the sag or separation by lifting or arching or otherwise shyly controlling the exposure.

The documentary circus will film anything. Anyone and everyone is encouraged and rewarded. The niggers respond on any cue.

You could fill the little child's head with all sorts of ideas. Not even physically rape it. Just tell it how bad its situation is; what it's missing, what it would be if it just had the breaks, the right amount of cash, the right strength, the right body.

Let it get through that phase of wanting to kill its captor. Let it decide that absolutely anything would be better than this.

Make it do it itself. Himself. Herself.

Let's make it herself.

"An 8-year old girl was raped after her mother traded her to a man for crack, police in Bossier City, LA, said."
(GIRL, 8, RAPED IN 'TRADE', *Chicago Sun-Times*, April '96)

"Cain told police Hill gave him the girl with the understanding he would have sex with her in exchange for crack, Halpin said. Police were alerted when workers at a local motel called them about the child."
(MOM CHARGED WITH SELLING GIRL FOR CRACK, *Chicago Tribune*, April '96)

What is a pig?

What does pig taste like, exactly?

How does pig suck, what does pig eat and how does pig grow into sex?

Just like it smells.

Just like you knew it would, when you thought about it, before you even took it, saw it, tasted it, fucked its fist before raping its tiny mouth and cunt with fingers and asshole days and days later when you just couldn't wait any longer.

How soon do you want to eat, honey?

How would you like to eat, dear?

I have to fucking listen to this mess.

Every fiber of its corpus is known to you before you summed up its technique, needs, what it was after the way it slurped and licked then sucked and dropped and deep throated to impress like some wheelchair bloated safed fuck would want to.

Here's your one and only chance.

Let it try to draw you in. To convince you. Fool you. This pig tastes like it talks, like you knew it would. She's a very sensitive pig.

She's just a cripple. She is a whole fucking cripple. This is her life, her stamp. Her brain swimming in halves. And the young dirty toxic fed baby becomes a cripple; her back breaks, her knees deform due to lack of proper exercise and care and as she grows she grows bent. Crooked cunt with glazed eyes focused on whatever my hand holds which is most often my cleansing pissing showering cock.

The cripple comes from the line that includes brain damaged wrecks pulled from their blood spattered metal car wrecks and ones that fell from high rise concrete out of thin holey gray window screens and the ones that slid the wrong way out of dysgenic cunts like the one she now holds so warm and dear and unloved. Which is why she cares.

Or at least, why she has to.

She lowers herself down unto any cock anywhere after all that baggage has been unhooked and unfastened and folded and cracked and screwed and broken, and all that baggage just drools and drips over me. Fat ugly cunt looking for a little fun. A better show. Mardi Gras friendly push and face make-up and a hideous, hideous lifelong disease.

Nipples so dark red and thickly pruned they belong to the baboon she mimics when she squats, fingers and plucks your cock from inside her fat asshole back to her hung open like a sore cunt.

Venereal disease could have caused those malformations. Some fucking disease could have crawled up inside you when you were drunk, or pretending to be, and you let it happen to you.

I like the way your sentence stops. The way you know how to talk – how to think and speak English perfectly well until you get to the word: AIDS. That word, those initials that step down so hard on your little blank head and choke your wind pipe and turn your face stupid and flush. I suck off those images right out of you: an autopsy room, a mother and her boyfriend being told by you on the phone and all the phoney play acting about what you're all going to do now when you know it is all about you. Only. And your decisions becoming choices less and less and your necessities becoming less and less demanding and less obvious and hardly important, now, in the face of things. And that image of you letting it into your body. So skinny and happy and dog content: bent over or ass high or tongue extended or face plastered flat, fist clenched, teeth grit, stomach tight, ass loose, cock hard, blood soaked, sweat wet and watery shit all sloshing down your thighs and sore hole as you get up too quick off the bed, table, floor, cloud. Back to you. Cunt. Faggot. Right back to that face. That smell of dirt in your body, on your palm, in your mouth. That cheese stink, that heavy cum, that hurtful body odor and the truth of memory and recognition and prepubescent focus.

It's not just the glory hole faggots acting like available women or the cripples pretending they're human or the children not knowing. It's not the system that sells female bodies as worthwhile or the whores who don't understand the marketplace.

Who wants to see a pair of tits or a cunt or a face waiting for a blow-job?

Some fatty Thai cunt – older than you'd expect or prefer – lies flat on her dead fluid staining back in a small swamp of green plants and grass and rich black mud, surrounded by thick black flies and crawling black ants. Her legs are spread wide in rape. Her fatty tits are flopped hung to each side of her gas bloated grey dead flesh chest. Naked death; her face sits straight up, mouth open, teeth hammered and raw.

Cops and technicians flit around her corpse as the cameraman floods the area patch with garish artificial light. A small Thai cop places a large green leaf over the raped gaping out and sunken vagina to prevent necessary digitising censorship later.

There are more close ups of another body, slice wounds that separate the skin into meaty chunks, red and yellow bubbled fat and scraped bone exposed inside the slashes thick and fist heavy. Bugs crawl over the body and around the cuts and dried scratching blood. Her black hair is matted and oily in gore and dirt and filth. Her face is torn into pieces; her teeth exposed wide as if she were mad and chomping open. Her eyes squished and closed tight.

Chop scars on her breasts, in between the cleavage and down the middle, boldly leaving the nipples clean and untouched.

My favorite is a little white girl laying in a squatted prone position, ass slightly up, head buried down and to its right side onto the floor, crammed right up next to a bed. Her baby brother is lying elsewhere on another bed with a large steel skinny poker imbedded and jutting straight up out of its tiny lunged chest. The baby's neck is viciously slashed open and pulled out. The little girl – I'm bad at guessing ages, but very young maybe 5 or 6 or 7 I hope – is barely clothed in tight pink underwear made sheer and disintegrating and tattered from the blood and piss and fecal shock. Her gentle dead ass cheeks pushed almost out sexily straight see through. A sleeping striped small t-shirt of pink and dirty white clads the upper half of her tiny titless torso and back. Her leg extends out uncomfortably as in a struggle from the rest of her compact death. Her thigh white clean peach meaty with just a few blood spatterings and pink scratches.

Blood is everywhere. The bathroom was filmed completely covered in it. And the toilet; thick pools and large splashes and, most importantly, these long dried sloshing drags where something, someone, had to splatter and spread it around in a liquid running mess.

The soundtrack is all in Japanese.

All you have is the pictures.

"Figure 8-46. Two sisters, ages 4 and 7 years, were raped and mutilated by their mother's live-in boyfriend. He killed the mother and left them all for dead. The children survived and identified their attacker. The older child (A through G), after the rape, was slashed several times with a knife. The knife was run, midline from below the anus, through the perineum and into the vagina. (A) Before surgery; (B) just before the surgery. She sustained a puncture

wound to her arm (C and D), a small laceration to her mid-chest (E), a laceration of her left arm (F), and defense wounds of her left hand where she tried to ward off her attacker (G). It is important to note that the palm wounds can be abuse injuries because children often defend themselves palm outward against their attackers. The younger child (H and I) had a knife slash across her throat (H) and evidence of anal abuse (I). She probably suffered the same abuse as her mother, who was anally penetrated with a broom handle. Compare the vaginal injury in the older child with cases of accidental injury, specifically with the child doing the splits and the child impaled on a light fixture (Figures 8-47 and 8-48)."
(CHILD MALTREATMENT; A COMPREHENSIVE PHOTOGRAPHIC REFERENCE IDENTIFYING POTENTIAL CHILD ABUSE, J.A. Monteleone, G. W. Medical Publishing, 1994.)

"FIGURE 8-82. This 3-year old boy was seen in the emergency room after complaining to his mother of anal pain. He disclosed anal penetration by his father. Note the increased pigmentation, funnelling, and moderate dilation. These are all nonspecific findings of abuse. With the history given, assuming that it is credible, they become stronger."
(CHILD MALTREATMENT; A COMPREHENSIVE PHOTOGRAPHIC REFERENCE IDENTIFYING POTENTIAL CHILD ABUSE, J.A. Monteleone, G. W. Medical Publishing, 1994.)

"FIGURE 9-11. This 9-year-old boy told a schoolteacher that he was chained at home.

Police investigators found him with a chain around his neck. The dog in the foreground was running free."
(CHILD MALTREATMENT; A COMPREHENSIVE PHOTOGRAPHIC REFERENCE IDENTIFYING POTENTIAL CHILD ABUSE, J.A. Monteleone, G. W. Medical Publishing, 1994.)

"FIGURE 9-12. Child punished with a cigarette lighter."
(CHILD MALTREATMENT; A COMPREHENSIVE PHOTOGRAPHIC REFERENCE IDENTIFYING POTENTIAL CHILD ABUSE, J.A. Monteleone, G. W. Medical Publishing, 1994.)

"FIGURE 3-7. Genital lesions that are abusive. This 5-year-old retarded child had penile narrowing below the glans (A and B) believed to be due to a stricture. The caregiver was trying to control the boy's bed-wetting."
(CHILD MALTREATMENT; A COMPREHENSIVE PHOTOGRAPHIC REFERENCE IDENTIFYING POTENTIAL CHILD ABUSE, J.A. Monteleone, G. W. Medical Publishing, 1994.)

"FIGURE 3-10. Flame burn of the penis that was believed to be caused by a cigarette lighter (A and B)."
(CHILD MALTREATMENT; A COMPREHENSIVE PHOTOGRAPHIC REFERENCE IDENTIFYING POTENTIAL CHILD ABUSE, J.A. Monteleone, G. W. Medical Publishing, 1994.)

"FIGURE 8-3. This 7-year-old girl described digital penetration. With labial separation the examination is not remarkable (A). The tear, at

nine o' clock, is seen after labial traction."
(CHILD MALTREATMENT; A COMPREHENSIVE PHOTOGRAPHIC REFERENCE IDENTIFYING POTENTIAL CHILD ABUSE, J.A. Monteleone, G. W. Medical Publishing, 1994.)

"The videos offered by Overseas Male were 'in actuality videotaped evidence of a crime taking place,' Hunter said. 'They show images of children having sex with each other or with adults – children as young as 7, 8 or 9 years old being sexually abused in unthinkable ways.'"
(POSTAL SERVICE STING TARGETS CHILD-PORN BUYERS, NETS 45, *Chicago Tribune*, May 19, 1996.)

"One of those arrested, Robert H. Ellison, pleaded for the return of several of his videos because he feared that he would molest children if he couldn't relieve his sexual urges through pornography, said Leo Lalley, a U.S. postal inspector.
    (...)Also arrested, on Oct. 25, 1995, was Samuel Bigknife, 44, of Niles. Lalley said a search of his home turned up newspaper articles on John Wayne Gacy and Jeffery Dahmer, as well as drawings of castration and decapitations."
(MAIL STING CAUGHT KID-PORN BUYERS, *Chicago Sun Times*, May 10, 1996.)

"I reflected on the injustices of the day. They had held me against my will for ten and a half hours, abused me, searched my home, damaged it (no telling what they had taken from it), confiscated my car and one of my trucks, all without even showing me a search

warrant or leaving a copy of it at the house – all over a missing kid who I didn't know, or see, and about whom I could not provide a scrap of help."
(A QUESTION OF DOUBT, John Wayne Gacy, Myco Associates, 1993.)

"WELCOME TO PRAGUE, THE CITY OF MANY ANGELS. 'NOT ANGELS BUT ANGELS' is a documentary about boy prostitution in Prague. The economic boom and the recently won political freedom have turned the beautiful, graceful city into a new mecca for both Eastern and Western tourists in search of sex. Young men trying to live up to the standards of Western consumerism readily fall prey to quick, easy money from hustling.
    The young hustlers' disarming frankness and need to talk become the compelling engine that drives this film. They withhold nothing. Rather they speak of their lives in often gruesome and stripped bare details, leaving us chilled by their short and fragile lives in the grasp of the oldest trade on earth."
(NOT ANGELS, BUT ANGELS, directed by Wiktor Grodecki, 80 minutes, Water Bearer Films, 1994.)

"But it was clear from comments by both a mother and one boy that both children had been involved in similar animal torture before, although both claimed the other was the instigator. During the interviews the mother and boy described incidents in which one goose was burned to death and a duck's nest was looted."
(BOYS' TORTURE OF GOOSE SHOCKS COUNTY

COURT, *Chicago Tribune*, April 30, 1996.)

"FIGURE 9-9. This 13 year-old boy stated that his father, while pinning the boy to the floor with his foot on the child's head, had beat him with a fishing rod numerous times. A neighbor noticed the marks on the boy's back (A and B) and reported it to the police. The father admitted to hitting the boy with a switch that was a three-foot section of fiberglass fishing rod."
(CHILD MALTREATMENT; A COMPREHENSIVE PHOTOGRAPHIC REFERENCE IDENTIFYING POTENTIAL CHILD ABUSE, J.A. Monteleone, G. W. Medical Publishing, 1994.)

"But prosecutors said evidence of the rape was overwhelming. It included a pubic hair found in the girl's diapers, which, when subjected to DNA testing by the Illinois State Crime lab, conformed to Pulfer's profile."
(90 YEAR TERM FOR INFANT'S RAPE, MURDER, *Chicago Tribune*, April 1996.)

"Police said Kenneth Hansen picked up the three boys on Oct. 16, 1955, as they hitchhiked home from a day roaming the city, going to a movie and two bowling alleys. Kenneth Hansen drove them to a stable on Chicago's Northwest Side, sexually abused them, strangled them and later dumped their bodies in a forest preserve ditch, police said."
(FORMER STABLEHAND DENIES TO SON THAT HE KILLED 3 BOYS IN 1995, *Chicago Tribune*, August 17, 1994.)

"FIGURE 8-61. This 12-year-old boy, along with his younger brother, described several episodes of anal penetration. Note the small anal tag at 11 o'clock and the venous defect at 1 o'clock. The younger brother had no physical findings suggestive of sexual abuse."
(CHILD MALTREATMENT; A COMPREHENSIVE PHOTOGRAPHIC REFERENCE IDENTIFYING POTENTIAL CHILD ABUSE, J.A. Monteleone, G. W. Medical Publishing, 1994.)

The cows are looking for encouragement. Empowerment. A new way to look at yourself, girls, regardless of the way others look, or leer, at you. Males. And the money these pricks wave, and the cocks they point, and the daughters or dirt they'd just as quickly fuck, don't matter when you close your eyes and float off to anywhere outside the sewer you call home.
    The cunts that judge them. The ones that don't understand your failure to conform is born of inability and just plain bad luck. Natural beauty passed some of us by. Outsider status is forced not selected. Chattel are born.
    The dregs collect. Seek and buy their level. And the mirror gets too crowded too quick. So full of fat used and sickly stupid cunts that there's no room for even one reasoning finger. One finger to prod its way between the slithering amassed cellulite and cancer and fading tattoos, the hormonal hair and early mother scar mistakes and yeast and boils and pits and fear and boredom and loneliness, and gently, so as not to startle or suddenly frighten such sensitive spirits, and point to the room at the back where their customers are

waiting.

The ones with money. The motherfuckers with control. The ones with eyes that don't see the womanly glow of acceptance and tantric time chakras. The ones who want to fuck a hole someday and have settled for what they can afford. The ones that close their eyes and pretend those thick spider varicose blue and green and red veins aren't there and don't matter until the next day when they think about how low they've sunk. The ones that maybe fuck with their eyes wide fucking open and take exactly what is on offer: Let's fuck a beast wrapped in lies and daddy pain. Let's fuck some hole who's only chance in life was to market the fat tits she sprouted when she was thirteen and now won't admit to their sagging or, rather, builds a new religion out of responding to the only attention she ever got and tried to keep that way.

The defensive fibs slowly contrived and meted out mock passionately is what the new mouth sells. The cricks and slits around the old mouth no longer used for blow-jobs is a powerful selling point in her hard won honesty. Her sister hole.

The words aren't merely naive or slanted, they are childish fantasies that hold to ignorance like a raped retarded girl in a packed court room answering, loudly, "NO" when asked by a defense attorney if, in fact, she is retarded.

Wilful in protection. Only.

Words that squish out to convince that only a sex negative asshole would say words that mean whores are receptacles for desperate people's hatred, anger and disease. Only a red neck frightened by his own sexuality, or lack thereof, or by general or size-specific inadequacy would see the flowery accepting advocacy of "Whores Heal" as incorrect readings of ideas as base as Whores Drip, Whores Stretch A Lot, and Whores Glaze Over.

 Excuses of this kind are formed of desperate clawing confusion stemming from finding yourself where you don't want to be but having done it for so long that the rot can only be prettied up not removed or hidden.

 Say you get home one evening and you're not filthy with drink and stupidity. You're not medically altered and the smell of your hands and clothes isn't redolent with tequila or poppers or pot. You're finely aware of your business.

 Few holes are so clearly homosexual.

 The mouth that sucked so tightly; like the wall itself was sucking all of you into that little fucking flesh pulled hole. Those tongue flicks tell you. The drags down the sides and length of what you feel of hard cock skin pulled tight.

 I can't tell if it's fists or his mouth until I pull out and see how soaking wet my hard beating red cock is. When I bend down to see what he wants more of, his fat tongue is extended into the lower clip of the wood. His face is a shivering panting wanting begging mouth hole: Dog faggot face with his trusting tongue lolling down against his lower lip wiggling it at me.

 He's tooling himself off, in there, on his knees, naked from the waist down except for his faggy hippy DMs and white rolled sports socks.

 His mouth is replaced by his muscled firm man butt that he grinds into the wood wall. He must feel his asshole in perfect position to the hole I look at. Spreads his ass cheeks and pushes the black open hole and beginning of his hanging hairy balls at me. Shit, motherfucker, come on shit. Big dark black crack and hairy stink and sweat matted caucasian flesh.

    This is a good idea. This is healthy. The worst thing that could happen to you in this far too short life is that you could live it fooled. And worse than that: that you could choose to live it that way.

    I push into his guts.

    Before someone would have wanted a condom or given me that look to come over there or go home with him.

    He wants it through the wood. And now. And sweaty. And pumping and slamming right into and through that fucking wall.

    I can smell his stink of amyl buzzing his thoughts and need and turning everything into just now.

    I cum into his asshole quick enough. And he knows it because he quits bucking and making so much fucking noise in a public place. The spasms in my cock are straight and staid and all the way in.

    He is death. He wants to reinfect. He slides off, a large wad of mucous cum sweated thin shit drips onto the cum and chlorine stinking floor from the tip of my pisshole and the edge of his asshole.

    His dog mouth cleans it up.

    He takes in his own AZT.

    We have guys who come in to lick the cum off the floor.

    He comes in here two or three times a day sometimes. At least once a day every day of the week no matter what, but he comes back a lot too.

    I'm told he's got a huge big dick that fills up the entire hole. He just can't get enough. He asks sometimes for ten dollars in quarters.

    That cocksucker that ate your body and

swallowed all sorts of new doses and toxins is a wife batterer, you're told by the fat black lump that smells behind the counter selling tokens and change and copies of swingers ads and few enough videos now and then.

The over the counter magazines have women spreading their legs and their meated cunts have been painted with lipstick. Like their mouths. Like targets. Hung out and kept that way with glue.

The cops actually came in here looking for him. So his wife knows what he does.

He told me he gets drunk and beats her. And sometimes he gets carried away and she calls the cops.

I know what fantasy is. I know full well how important it is to define reality and not be fooled, not to be lulled into laziness and empty safety. I know the difference between fake and actual dreams and wishes, hope and need. I know what I want and what I've had.

I know I can't feel the fists he fucks his wife with when he pulls me off through his side of the wall. The mouth that spits at that stupid white trash whore that wraps around my cock and licks on the thick main vein that pushes into his face could be anyone's.

But it isn't.

Do you have any children? I asked him finally.

I want to know if you fuck your children.

Do you suck off your child; your little boy? Do you fuck his ass?

I let him lick my balls. I gave him some dick. I jerked myself off asking him questions while he stared at me.

You like big dick?

Does your wife suck cock like you?

I want to know how old your boy is and what he looks like in the bathroom being fed your drunk dick smelling like all the mouths in here.

Do you beat your child?

Do you fucking abuse your baby boy?

It's better than fucking cunts isn't it?

This cunt will talk on and on about the power of pussy if you let it. About how he fell in love with vaginas when he first got a glimpse in, what, grade school and how he's been hooked ever since.

This puffed faggot will convince himself that cunt – fucking females – is somehow worthy of talking about, about spending time working out the peculiarities of his attraction and the strength he possesses in, first, giving into the natural drive and second, his forthrightness in detailing his daily dip.

How he fucks cunt. How he talks at it and has come to protect it and his overburdened need for it.

There's these little morons; these little bugs scurrying around in circles crackling their little holes and clicking out tiny scraping noises over which wet little ads sound: I fuck cunt. I take care of my children. Why not pick on someone your own size.

And the State will take care of the bills for your next child born with a hole in its retarded rat heart.

And all the cum that slid down your wife's hideous barking throat and around the decaying walls of her womb is tinted with reason and desire and nature's will.

And love is what you own when you tend to your package. Love is the idea that lies under you when you stand arm and arm at the welfare office thinking about all the cunt it fucks and the little diseases it protects and how snugly excuses fit into the big comfortable black hole that is that bleeding chewed vagina and his jerking off in front of the TV set.

I know fags who say the same thing.

You fuck cunt, you suck cock. You beat a cock off with your greasy fist wrapped around it, your open soaked hanging lips pressed and rubbing up against the fat purple cock head, other hand working the space between ball sac and asshole. Someone, anyone tonight, comes into that hole. You feed that hole. You pump and grind into that faggot's face and feel that tongue and that pressure, that relief, that easy focus on just one clear idea, one all warm busy idea like nature and anger and need and want and you cum into that face that works around you. Or that cunt that flops its tits into your face. And it thinks: I love cunt. Or ass. Asshole. Hairy man's ass sucking up the sweat with a hand towel that your wife cleans her make-up off with.

You should find what it is you want.

Your child is probably waiting at home now thinking the exact same thing.

Ask what he wants. Show him what you know.

I fucking know you wouldn't tell the beast at the front that you beat your little boy. Or better: fucked his shit all in and showed him how you sucked my cock.

I understand. You can tell me.

I want to know.

I tore up my garbage into little pieces. The cops tried to put them together. It makes perfect sense to me to look to what's already legal for your pleasures.

A video exists of a couple burly looking Portuguese speaking greaseballs holding down a young boy. There's a few men running about on camera arguing and shouting. The camera moves from the argument – heated sweating apes yelling close to each other's faces – and into a crowd quickly forming around the youth.
    The camera points down directly at the frightened dark-yellowish face of the boy. His eyes wide and darting, his struggle and fear and helplessness clear and contorted on his biting South American ghetto features. Big shoulders and fat fingers knock into the camera and add confusion to the violence. It is quite probable that the arguing is just over the camera being present.
    A large blue denim shirt sleeve with a big dark brown hairy hand gropes a small black rusty pistol and, almost as soon as it appears pointing down at the boy, the camera is jostled – forcibly pulled back. Quick faces with beards and a brick wall fuzz by and blur later on pause. The camera is brought back down amid a large laugh and tries to recapture its previous focusless aim.
    The boy has already been turned over. The camera was jumped not by the thugs, it seems, but rather by the aggressive flip of the boy face down into the concrete. The frame is shaky and nervous and amateur intensive, and the pistol cracks, like quick pops, two right on top of each other, happen far too fast for any emotional connection. The boy's slick black hair is immediately blacker from the red and all the yelling stops as the camera is quickly pointed to a wall and turned off. The image that stays was just all wet hair and blood just starting to

fan out onto hard concrete against his flattened face, one would guess.

I would have preferred to see the boy laid flat on his back, the gun shoved deep into his mouth like a cock rape and the trigger pulled right next to his dirty hard teeth. A huge pool of blood faucets out on the alley beneath his exploded head and the men who held him down can't help but get their big black boots wet in it. They leave large footprints and thick red streaks as they move abruptly over his body and, disturbed by the mess and now the evidence, the last one to let go of the lifeless skinny young arms and torso starts to kick it with his bloody boot. The boy's dead face then comes closer into focus to display his smashed jagged front teeth, sunken and collapsed eyes and nose bridge and cheekbones: the skull inside his face being shattered from the gun blast he sucked off last.

I would like to see the camera turned off then only after seeing, maybe, his plastic baggy filled and burnt with glue. Or it would have been best to have had the killers come across the boy as he was head down huffing, his eyes slits and oily dark bad complexion black heads on deep tan wasted teenage skin all glazed over and chemical dead. They should have humiliated him, or tried to; given his extreme brain drugged state. Pulled down his loose pants and slapped his numb face to make his thin pointy flaccid Brazilian uncut dick wiggle and bounce lifeless. They should have put the boot in there. And stuck the gun into his dry asshole, fucked him with that little tube gun barrel just as an idea, a symbol, rather than the pain that would have most probably been lost on the zombie anyways. Blowing his guts out of his shithole or shooting his cock off or more boot kicking and hard fist punching would have taken the video out of its utilitarian state and placed it firmly into the sexual. These brutish Brazilian thugs who have to do a job, basically have to dispatch any number of these street thieve urchins, could've enjoyed themselves much more. Taken advantage of their position and rarefied good fortune. The boy died anyway. And too fucking quickly.

It's what I saw, what I liked about it and then what it meant to me. What I think the implications are and the reality that is formed by that information. Where it pointed to in my fantasies, my desires and tastes. What the lame fucks missed.

A rat brown haired female mess in loose grey sweat pants and a large thick winter t-shirt with what looks like a hand painted bunny swinging on a swing on the front is filmed talking to someone in the front seat of a car. It's still light out, possibly early afternoon even, and her dirty sweats are easily glimpsed in her slump and the light. The car must be somewhere secluded though. The car is in park, the radio going, some beating noise, the driver holding the camera and leaning, must be, up against the door. The driver's white rough hand reaches out into the tight frame and pets the white trash's breast over the t-shirt, then down over her belly making a large arc motion whereby it quickly becomes obvious that this daytime whore is very pregnant. The hand on the shirt flattens the palsy painted homey shirt against a vary taut protuberance that seems far too round to be just fat. The woman lurches forward into the camera and starts to fiddle with where the driver's belt and zipper must be. Almost as immediately the driver's back straightens out, arches a little and the lens is pointed to the nest of hair in his lap. All the frame becomes, because of the position of the driver and the compactness of the car, is her head -her ratty hair- bobbing up in anyone's lap and nothing more. Surely that cock remains soft in her anxious head. She is far too quick and no genitalia or mouth can be seen. The steering wheel is actually pushing up against her hair and if she becomes too aggressive or lost in her performance, she's sure to bang her high forehead on the way up or down that dick.

    This turns out to be just a taste. Perfunctory. Establishing shot. The camera is turned off and the edit clipped to a quilted orange and brown covered small bed snuggled tight into a badly wall-papered corner. The pregnant beast now sits on the bed with her squat legs across the width of the bed and her hurting back against the wall. Her pregnant lap sinking into the dilapidated mattress springs.

    She is somewhat toothless when she opens her mouth to small talk; therefore a crackwhore. She doesn't smile when she asks the cameraman if she should strip and doesn't wait for an answer. She seems to be announcing it more than anything else. She lifts that shirt off in a clumsy bend and pulls and lumps back to the wall to show her firm rock hard pregnancy tits jutting just above a smooth dimestore lamp light reflecting round child twisting belly. Her jogging pants actually continue to cover the lower portion of her pregnant sag and she shifts her ass up just a little, the slightest effort necessary certainly, and wrests the dirty old material off by tugging it in clumps at her knees.

    She picks in the hair between her varicose legs and on top of her head, absent mindedly, but suddenly exposed and vulnerable. She's left her cheap laundry room sneakers on. Steeling herself in whatever drugged up way she can.

She leans up further against the wall and then slacks just a little; slumps her weight down to her neck and middle back to showcase her puffed in cunt for the camera. She finger slips the lips apart and spreads her pliable gummed meat flesh barely open: gristled and brownish and blotchy red and disgusting wirey brown dark rat's fur hair pushing and curling and twisting every which way inside that rank whore's nest.

The frame again grows smaller, the objects larger, as the camera goes in for a close-up. Her face is glimpsed in a second before the focus is all gross cunt: teeth here and there in empty red sick gums all in the middle of her mouth, lipstick, lousy bumpy skin, eye shadow and blush and half mast heavy lidded genetic stupidity.

The frame expands and pans up the hair trickling from her pubic mound like ants up her belly to her puckered and pregnant deformed navel. Her dark reddish almost brown wrinkled mother's nipples and a large pink pus yellow zit on her tit. Her face again bored and uncaring and, even, unaccommodating. She wants to let the camera idiot fuck her and get it over with.

Her position shifts in a shaky moment as she lays down further on the bed and seems to grab his dick at the same time. The camera's voice telling her to wait. He's gotta "work on it a minute first."

These are the first two scenes of four that matter. The rest is all humping. The camera is placed on a tripod a little too far from the bed and as the john – now pot bellied, balding and somewhat withered with a fat but short stubby cock that's hard immediately – checks continually to a monitor just off screen it seems. He fucks her gaseous cunt as she lays flat back on the bed; their bellies slapping, one tight and hard, the other flabby and loose, and stopping each other as his arms carry his weight above her shoulders. She sucked him a little. And a little more when he pulls out of her pruned cunt and mounts her face, obscuring almost everything with pregnant belly and his fleshy ass cheeks. He finally jerks himself off, like most videos with pregnant pigs, all over her stomached fetus and tits. While she just lays there flat and waits for the wipe.

The final two edits are complementary. She sits, clothed again, on the bed and talks to the cameraman who is again holding the camera up to his eye. She's drinking from a small wash glass that she immediately relaxes into. She pours back into the glass from a green bottle of Tanqueray gin. She's also smoking a cigarette and portrays proper bar style with cigarette and gin all in one hand. The talk is clear and boring; mostly about how long she had to wait for someone both of them know to show up for a ride somewhere.

Then she raises her shirt to show her monster gut naked and says: "This'll work for ya."

She stubs the end of her lit cigarette out on her belly. The other hand holding the gin up high in wait. She doesn't make a sound or a wince. It seems the act is more gesture than burn, though the butt does crumble beneath the stub evincing some dedication to purpose.

"You don't want the baby?"
"I don't know the baby."
"You don't like it?"
"I don't know it. I don't like bein'

pregnant."

The cameraman gets up from where he's been sitting and close-ups on the belly mark. Just grey ash, no puffiness or pink hurt.

Another edit replaces what should have been more conversation and focus.

The new frame is filled with her pregnant to filled up pigness and bursting belly. Her navel is down at the bottom of the screen, a single tit just at the top right. It doesn't look so polished even in the reflected light, though rather blotchy and unevenly pricked and pimpled. Much less clean and perfect and more troubled and manhandled.

The cameraman's dirty fingers stub out another cigarette on the middle of the bloated stomach. She flinches and burps out a small squeal. He grinds it into her skin and rubs out the orange burn across the sickening baby weight.

Nothing is said but she continues to moan a little bit extra.

A third cigarette, that must have been lit at the same time as the second, is put out on her mothered existence just as quickly as he can manipulate the shaky camera and his fingers. This one drooled sparks down her round belly that may have fallen unto the bed or her pubic nest. She twitches less, having been prepared for it but almost bounces herself forward. She sort of whistles and says it hurt a little more that time.

"Little motherfucker," the cameraman says for some reason.

"Yeah," she says and the tape ends in ash smear close up.

He could have asked her when she was due. He could have put the cigarettes out inside her cunt and lit matches underneath the nipples the little crack addicted head bursting quivering mess needs to suckle at. He could have smashed the Tanqueray bottle against a table and shoved the glass shards into her cunt: to hurt her and make her bleed. To offer a jagged cutting pathway for the baby to crawl and die through. He could have performed a C-section right there and then and beat the pregnant pig to slow bone snapped, drug pulled death with a baseball bat. Smashing down on the baby belly womb. Smashing down on it so it collapses and fells and expels. Breaking the ribs that spread. Breaking the tendons and fluid pouches and feed veins into pulp and all the little forming soft vermin break and bend cat bones.

I know why I bought the video. I know what I'm looking for. And I know what they're playing with.

Let all the edges be blurred with money. Let the beasts involve themselves in filth and rationalize their positions with the need of finance. I know what a job is. I know what a mess reality is. I don't want to fuck it. I want to support it and encourage and exploit and silently control. Let them live and breathe and collect and think.

I know what they do and what they offer. I know what I clean up and purchase. What I display, move and hide.

He should have asked her:
How long have you been drinking?
When is the baby due – do you know, have you gone for a sonogram, did you worry about whether or not to get an abortion?
Have another drink.
Do you know who any of the fathers will be?
Are you still addicted to crack?

Can I buy you a rock? Can I film you blasting your face with your homemade pipe and plastic bottle, naked, pregnant, puffed and burning, feeling fucked and alive and filthy and mothered and motherly again?

Will you be around to hold your shivering baby if it's born addicted to crack? From what I understand, that's what those little packages of born pain desire most – just to be held. How d'ya think the doctors know that?

Will they let you breast feed? What do you lactate?

Do you have a regular doctor? A favorite, comfortable clinic stop?

What has a doctor said about your bruises and teeth?

You have to fucking tell them, don't you? You can fucking talk to them, can't you, because you fucking have to, right?

Do you understand what's going on?
Do you know what you're doing?
Can you care?
What you are?
What you're selling?
What I'm buying?

He should have explained to her that the video need only be for him, but she had no control either way.

And he had every intention of selling it to me and specific others, anyways.

And that he bought her. All of her. Twenty minute flat back fuck and the pregnant disgust and car blow-job through crack teeth face all for sale. And it's all she has left. To offer. Always.

The reality is mine. Her entire daily life and whatever makes her smile, cum or forget is in my pocket – when I pull out the cash to pay and when I put the video back in. Her half an hour of life is all I want. Let her go back to her mundane density and morning sickness, her plans to raise a garden sometime, or another kid, or finish a class in real estate. Let her hide her tampon and pull out her whiskers here and there; let her call her mom or get one nice dinner a week or an early morning cup of coffee or a nice shit: it's all garbage to me. It's all here clean and real in a half an hour and, at the same time exactly, all that I want and all she has to sell. I watch it again and again and hope to fucking hell she's abused into the hard black dirt again and again every fucking time I watch it with my hard-on cumming all over my fist and cheap holed underwear.

  I'm interested, honey, in everything you are.
  Because I own every bit of your reality.
  And I own all of them. As somewhere right now there's some stupid girl pitching in to help around a punk rock club and working nights at a rape crisis center. And she used to be a stripper and had cum after cum splashed into her glass frozen face just like the rape she slid through when she was fifteen. And this little ignorant darling supports me. Keeps the place open for me. Hands out rubbers to whores for me to cum in and puts her shoulder out for the ones I want to rape – want to: see everyday: ain't no nigger – and sells it all right back to me. Time and time again.

  You lost honey. As soon as you see yourself included in the group, you lost the big war. As soon as you think your acts help those behind or below you; all of femalia, you just joined the ranks. You sick condescending monkey on a stick. You cheap titted dancer for men. You moron in make-up and roller skates.

Bad mistake.

Someone's got to teach you.

How to stand up for yourself.

How to lose with dignity.

The correct way to go through someone's pocket while you're rubbing your tits in their face or on their cock. When your mouth is full of their balls, when you're speared onto their cock.

The right thing to do with your money. Easy money is too often easy spent, easy wasted.

You don't have to use drugs just like you don't have to let someone piss in your face. Or cum in your mouth.

You can remain in control.

It's just an image on the screen.

It's their problem, not yours.

I'll give you an example.

I'm not interested in the touch of someone else's flesh.

I'm not without insecurities. As I get older I see that many were warranted but I seem to care less. With every extra pound of weight I gain my cock seems to get smaller and deader. As I get older this is of some comfort to me. Let the niggers be niggers. I'm tired and lazy and I've become that hulk that the girls want to finish quickly and steal from. I look like a slave that doesn't know what he wants, who he's fooling or what he's getting. Fair enough, I figure, I'm in paying mode and I wish my cock was even smaller, my belly bigger, my need to keep clean more forgiving.

I thought paying one of the whores I was fucking in Japan for something other than their slippery thin pink long haired cunts might be a good idea. Every one of these prostitutes was exactly like any other cunt anybody has ever fucked. The look in their lidless eyes, the weight of their small boney laps, the slide of their existence on top or below me.

    She could move any way she likes. A barnyard pig. Weasel bait. A cummy model. A bored brat like a teen coked strawberry. Dead fish but not dead all the way. She could bark, giggle, try her English out retard style or talk porno. She could sit back and count her money as her tiny pug nose twitches out just the slightest quickest or most overpowering waft of cunt womb rotting menstrual yeast. I don't care how many men did or didn't cum into her. I don't give a fuck what she's going to put all her yen to. Her gossip. Her in-fighting. Her customer condescension. Her ideas and dreams and highest sale period. I don't want to think she has any opinion other than pure contempt for me. How she rationalizes her position, her situation, is entirely up to her.

    Her flat stomach, her soft bones, her make-up thicked pock marks and dull work eyes. Her copy of *Hit Parade*, *Vogue*, *Uomo* or some subway comic book. Her mexican flab. Her nigger lips. Black beef. Skinny slow cunt. Her slurred words or impolite refusal to speak, or admit she understands, English. Her asshole that closes tight to rosebud dark flesh or that mucous that circles the gaping distended pit that beats slack long after the cum has soaked into its intestines. Her muscleless mouth and tiny fingers. My anywhere from 20 to 200 dollar cock.

    This last one understood perfectly the price in yen. And that I didn't want her to use her hands or, most important, her neck or tongue.

    I thought just fucking its face was a better

idea this time. Using it like a stunted Japanese flesh bucket. A hole I fed in and out of, a brained up skull I fucked myself with.

Don't move your fucking tongue. Just open your mouth and leave it open like a dummy. Honestly, I won't choke you. I won't go too fast. I don't want to. Just open up and I'll fuck your black slick haired soft head.

I did this for awhile.

I wanted to take some of the kiddie porn I bought from the shop just down the corner from my hotel and look at it while I fucked this little burning paid-for face.

She was anybody.

She was flesh and a hooker who did this for, from what I understand, a rather acceptable living.

I could have had younger. More like the little growing into girls in the pictures I chose this time out, probably. Though I suspect the pornography is a much easier acquisition. I also could have had cheaper and more demeaned, more dejected and available. And it follows, there was a large selection of much higher priced smarter girls.

I didn't want to fuck the kind of girl in the pictures.

The youngest of whom, I'm guessing, was around six or seven. Quite young and full of long thick cock to lick and jerk off. A still or two from a film and some lovely polaroid reproductions from America.

This cunt whose head I gift wrapped my cock in could have, would have, dressed down to a school girl uniform and made like she didn't know what I, as the very old man, wanted from her just budding youth.

This has nothing to do with power.
She came in here sold.
This has nothing to do with my parents.
This has nothing to do with baby flesh.
This has nothing to do with hate or lust.
This has nothing to do with females.
I'm just visiting.
This is just what's available.
This is just what's on display.
This is within my price range.

    I had put her on her knees, onto the carpet in between the American style bed advertised and the desk against the wall. I faced the window with the drapes closed tight. I pumped into her face rhythmically, mechanically. I wasn't altering my thrusts or my interests. I held my hands at the sides of her face to keep her still and steady. A gently running breathing sewer. I put the magazine – color, digest sized, LOLITAPOP in large green letters on the cover above a thin shapeless torso cut at the nose and hairless pristine vagina, just at her straight thighs – directly on top of her black hair head and creased it as flat as I could. I only turned the pages twice or so. I settled eventually on a younger little girl lying flat on a bed, the camera at her feet towering over her while another man, the partner, stood at her head and lowered a long soft cock into her face. The girl's tongue inched out of her thin mouth just barely to touch the tip of the purple headed cut thick cock, his balls dangling in her soft blondish brown hair that, as she matured into just the first few years of teenage would probably turn dirty brown all on its own. The partner's one hand was reached out and tucked to put a finger into her bald flat surprisingly spread out cunt slash. Her legs might have looked better kept shut tight in fear. Natural fighting rape response. But the cameraman, no doubt, told her to spread. Do the fucking splits on your back. Her little eyes were unclear in the shot, just little dots when I stared too much breaking up the photo into printing technique and poor reproduction quality with a long history of sales, but I did wonder if she was looking at the camera man for instructions or to the balls and cock being hung down steadily into her short soft face.

 I had flipped through this magazine before. I had masturbated with it before. Sitting on my bed, with my back up and my cock perpetually hard as I stroked and kept teasing myself as I found a better image, a better image, a closer image than I expected every page I kept turning. Every magazine from the collection I was quickly gathering during my brief vacation.

 Another one. Flat chest, boned nothing nipples, a ten year old bud who's had make-up applied to her baby cocksucker face.

 Another one. With an engorged big cock stuffed into the beginning of its small stretched mouth and eye squint like she didn't like the taste of paste in school.

 Another one. A firm little ass spread wide open and bent over.

 The shot with someone's tongue pressed into that hole. Her baby asshole clean of stench and shit and now sullied with demands and money and trauma.

 Sat on a cock. The balls flattened against the thin roll-less weight of her white thighs and boy hips. Hairless; it fits perfectly up to all its brims.

 So much to choose. So many perfect shots. So many more to look through and then leave behind.

And this face I work into. Who doesn't care. Except for the money. That's what she sees instead of my hairy lumpy sac hanging old and slapping ever so rudely, steadily, gently onto her chin and supple Japanese neck. My cock in the back of its throat, sliding against that lifeless tasteless tongue, her teeth high and low in her breathing mouth absentmindedly but conscious of my hard hot skin and thick cabled vein and hair and stretched to pain spongy cock head.

I like this photo.

I like what happened.

The space between his cock and his fingers is just barely a foot or two, encompassing that child's entire body in its expanse. In his shadow. His intention. His reality. So compact is she. So small and sold and ready.

I paid this whore.

I paid for this magazine.

Bottom runging.

I know if I ejaculate into her mouth, she'll pull back in fear. I don't need an uncomfortable moment, not when this is what I worked up to.

I feel the sperm in my crotch collecting, I feel the cords in my spine arching, I feel my cock pursing and dribbling pre-cum.

I pull out and masturbate myself. Just once, twice, a few times hard quick strokes and juts, down my rather dry length into her face. The magazine is still on her head, she politely stays in place, rooted, naked little tits to the floor as I cum all over her chest and arms as I point down and she doesn't flinch, doesn't move away, keeps the magazine open to that little fingerfuck and blow-job tongue.

That little girl in the room with those two cocks. The cameraman had to have a piece. I'd like to see more shots, one after another, of what happened – pity this is a collection of scenes like the Japanese are so fucking fond of. I want to see more eyes. More fingers stuck in up there and more tongue and mouth.

More cocaine. More vomit that I don't smell or hide. That rains down on tears and bruises badly covered in wine and bad make-up to cut the glare.

I focused on the magazine, not the mouth. Not the head I fucked into. My dick slid in and out of someone else's life but I didn't even watch, couldn't see it and the fucking child getting raped up to some boney ring finger slosh and dig and dig.

Let them cum huge thick loads of white porno jism into that throat; down that open gullet and choking sold tears.

Sperm spills down from my pisshole. I stroke it clean. Let the cum dangle like snot, in long gelatinous globs that stretch and connect to her chest, Japanese tits with slightly brownish nipples being something of a purer breed, I suppose, and soak into the dust and dirt in the hotel carpet.

Lick it. Lick it, don't suck.

As my penis slowly grows soft, too quickly actually, as I hold it and start to drag my fingers into and around my sinking ball sac flesh, a couple of my fingers getting nice and close to my asshole. My thumb rooted against the heavy base of my pubic hair and cock.

Lick it and I'll pay you extra yen. I'll give you a tip. Bad pun.

She does. Cleans my cock. My AIDS. No long stem tongue drag and slurps. Just workman mouth swallows and envelope and cheeks drawn in to smack. Puts her head on it and dives in.

I like it flaccid and in her face. The magazine has been placed on the bed to the side. I keep my hands away from her head and let her do her job. This time. For awhile.

I move out clean. Mouth spit clean. All my cock stink is left on her tongue, I suppose, I hope. She'll draw it back into her mouth and swallowing air and spit she'll taste all of my money in her gut and retch. For her to take home. Or back to her closet or fixing room or wherever, like she always has done.

I could've had her move her head. Had a proper blow-job like she's been trained. I could've easily put the magazine on the bed and turned my head to it as she kept the same position. Turning the pages with one arm outstretched every now and again.

I could've instructed her to turn the page.

Stop sucking and find me a nice little damage.

I didn't need her head still. It's how I wanted it. I just wanted to fuck a face – her face, as it turned out. Her mouth, her head, her foreign existence and everyone she's ever known or been paid to be fucked by.

I, at that particular time, wanted that information. Next time I'll want anybody else. Next time I won't need a head at all. Next time I won't need the magazine.

Next time I won't be able to.

I just made my money work for me.

And I know what fantasy is, and what safety is, and what I did and what I paid and exactly what I got.

Next time I'll be breathing it all in.
This was no coveted moment. This was a part I purchased. I own all of her reality and the most interesting thing – the most amazing thing – for me is that she – that anybody – is completely immaterial.

www.creationbooks.com